HPNA PALLIATIVE NURSING MANUALS

Social Aspects of Care

Edited by

Nessa Coyle, PhD, APRN, FAAN

Consultant
Palliative Care and Clinical Ethics in Oncology
New York, New York

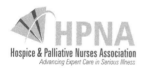

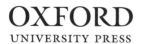

OXFORD
UNIVERSITY PRESS

Oxford University Press is a department of the University of
Oxford. It furthers the University's objective of excellence in research,
scholarship, and education by publishing worldwide.

Oxford   New York
Auckland   Cape Town   Dar es Salaam   Hong Kong   Karachi
Kuala Lumpur   Madrid   Melbourne   Mexico City   Nairobi
New Delhi   Shanghai   Taipei   Toronto

With offices in
Argentina   Austria   Brazil   Chile   Czech Republic   France   Greece
Guatemala   Hungary   Italy   Japan   Poland   Portugal   Singapore
South Korea   Switzerland   Thailand   Turkey   Ukraine   Vietnam

Oxford is a registered trademark of Oxford University Press
in the UK and certain other countries.

Published in the United States of America by
Oxford University Press
198 Madison Avenue, New York, NY 10016

© Oxford University Press 2016

Library of Congress Cataloging-in-Publication Data
Social aspects of care / edited by Nessa Coyle.
p. ; cm. — (HPNA palliative nursing manuals ; volume 6)
Includes bibliographical references and index.
ISBN 978–0–19–024413–2 (alk. paper)
I. Coyle, Nessa, editor.   II. Series: HPNA palliative nursing manuals ; v. 6.
[DNLM: 1. Hospice and Palliative Care Nursing. WY 152.3]
RA1000
362.17′56—dc23
2015023116

9 8 7 6 5 4 3 2 1
Printed in the United States of America
on acid-free paper

HPNA PALLIATIVE NURSING MANUALS

Social Aspects of Care

HPNA PALLIATIVE NURSING MANUALS

Series edited by: Betty R. Ferrell, RN, PhD, MA, FAAN, FPCN, CHPN

Contents

Preface

This is the sixth volume of a new series being published by Oxford University Press in collaboration with the Hospice and Palliative Nurses Association. The intent of this series is to provide palliative care nurses with quick reference guides to each of the key domains of palliative care.

Content for this series was derived primarily from the *Oxford Textbook of Palliative Nursing* (4th edition, 2015) which is also edited by Betty Ferrell, Nessa Coyle, and Judith Paice, the editors of this series. The contributors identified in each volume are the authors of chapters in the *Oxford Textbook of Palliative Nursing*, from which the content was selected for this volume. The Textbook contains more extensive content and references, so users of this Palliative Nursing Series are encouraged to use the Textbook as an additional resource.

We are grateful to all palliative care nurses who are contributing to the advancement of care for seriously ill patients and families. Remarkable progress has occurred over the past 30 years in this field and nurses have been central to that progress. Our hope is that this series offers an additional tool to build the care delivery system we strive for.

Contributors

Patricia Berry, PhD, RN, ACHPN, FAAN, FPCN

Professor of Nursing
Director, Hartford Center of
    Gerontological Nursing
    Excellence
School of Nursing
Oregon Health and Science
    University
Portland, Oregon

Inge B. Corless, PhD, RN, FAAN

Professor of Nursing
MGH Institute of Health
    Professions
Boston, Massachusetts

Betty Davies, RN, CT, PhD, FAAN

Adjunct Professor and Senior
    Scholar
School of Nursing
University of Victoria
Victoria, Canada

Julie Griffie, RN, MSN, ACNS-BC, AOCN

Manager, Nursing Practice
Clinical Cancer Center
Medical College of Wisconsin
Froedtert Hospital
Milwaukee, Wisconsin

Marianne Matzo, PhD, APRN-CNP, FPCN, FAAN

Professor and Frances E. and
    A. Earl Ziegler Chair in Palliative
    Care Nursing
Director of Sooner Palliative Care
    Institute
University of Oklahoma College of
    Nursing
Director of Survivorship and
    Supportive Care Center
Adjunct Professor of Geriatric
    Medicine
Peggy and Charles Stephenson
    Cancer Center
Oklahoma City, Oklahoma

Polly Mazanec, PhD, ACNP-BC, AOCN, FPCN

Assistant Professor
FPB School of Nursing
Case Western Reserve University
Cleveland, Ohio

Joan T. Panke, MA, APN, ACHPN

Palliative Consultant/Palliative
    Care NP
Arlington, Virginia

Rose Steele, RN, PhD

Professor of Nursing
York University
Toronto, Ontario, Canada

Chapter 1

Sexuality

Marianne Matzo

> ### Key Points
> - Sexuality is an integral part of the human experience.
> - Healthcare providers often overlook the sexual needs of those receiving palliative care.
> - Communication, privacy, and practical solutions to physical changes may have a positive impact on sexual health for the palliative care patient.

This chapter highlights sexuality as an important aspect of palliative care. Incurable illness and end-of-life care may compromise a couple's intimacy. To prevent or minimize this, healthcare practitioners should assume a leading role in the assessment and remediation of potential or identified alterations in sexual functioning. Not all couples will be concerned about their sexual health at this point of their life together. However, if sexual health is desired, all attempts should be made to facilitate this important aspect of life. People may find that being physically close to the one they love is life affirming and comforting.

As patients draw close to the end of life, their needs, hopes, and concerns remain intact as in any other stage of their life. Assessment of sexual health should occur for all patients to determine whether these needs and hopes include maintenance of their sexual health. The healthcare practitioner's offer of information and support can make a significant difference in a couple's ability to adjust to the changes in sexual health during end-of-life care.

Case Study: A Patient With End-Stage Ovarian Cancer

"I think that I prefer that at least I have information, so the more information I have at least I feel like I'm in control. I just remember that information about intimacy was very limited out there. You know, could you have sex, could you not? What was viable, what wasn't after surgery? Frankly, no one ever talked to me about that if you want to know the truth. Anything that I did find, I pursued it and looked for it, because it was a bullet point, or two or three in a brochure that was given to me by a nurse or a doctor or who ever. That's all I got, was a couple of bullet points, and that's really not enough."

Advanced illness and end-of-life care can interfere with sexual health and physical sexual functioning in many ways. These include physiological changes; tissue damage; other organic manifestations of the disease; attempts to palliate the symptoms of advancing disease, such as fatigue, pain, nausea, and vomiting; and psychological sequelae such as anxiety, depression, and body-image changes. The complexities of human sexuality are broad, especially for people coping with life-threatening illness and those who are facing the end of their lives. The sexual health model[1] (Figure 1.1) reflects these complexities by identifying ten broad components

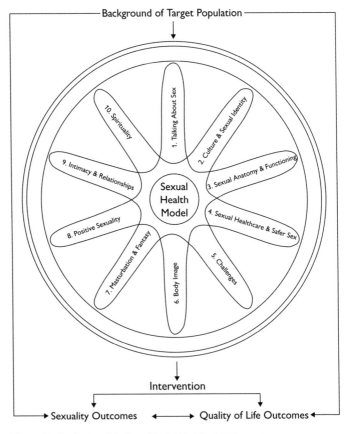

Figure 1.1 Application of the Sexual Health Model to HIV Prevention

From Robinson BBE, Bockting WO, Simon Rosser BR, Miner M, Coleman E. The sexual health model: application of a sexological approach to HIV prevention. Health Educ Res. 2002;17(1):43–57.

posited to be essential domains of healthy human sexuality: talking about sex; culture and sexual identity; sexual anatomy and functioning; sexual healthcare and safer sex; overcoming challenges to sexual health; body image; masturbation/fantasy; positive sexuality, intimacy and relationships; and spirituality and values.[1] An Institute of Medicine report that addresses cancer care for the whole patient states that, in order to ensure appropriate psychosocial health, healthcare practitioners should facilitate effective communication.[2] One study of an oncology population documented that 28% of the patients indicated their physicians do not pay attention to anything other than their medical needs.[3] This chapter is organized according to each component of the sexual health model.[1]

Talking About Sex

A cornerstone of the sexual health model is the ability to talk comfortably and explicitly about sexuality, especially one's own sexual values, preferences, attractions, history, and behaviors.[1] This communication is necessary to effectively express needs to a partner and to discuss with a healthcare provider the alterations in sexual health that have resulted from illness. Psychological distress that patients or their partners experience during diagnosis and treatment of malignancy can impair a healthy sexual response cycle.[4]

Culture and Sexual Identity

Culture influences one's sexuality and sense of sexual self. The cultural meaning of sexual behaviors needs to be taken into account, because that meaning may impact a person's willingness or interest in maintaining sexual intimacy while receiving palliative care. The patient and family are at the center of palliative care. A patient's desire or interest in maintaining physical sexual relations is highly variable. Some may find expression of physical love an important aspect of their life right up to death, while others may relinquish their "sexual being" early in the end-of-life trajectory. Each individual's identity is influenced, in part, by his or her sexual identity. Roles between spouses or sexual partners are additionally defined by the sexual intimacy between them. Sexual integrity can be both altered and compromised during the course of an incurable disease, deleteriously affecting both the identity and the role fulfillment of the affected person. Sexuality goes far beyond "sexual intercourse." Sexuality may encompass physical touch of any kind, as well as experiences of warmth, tenderness, and the expression of love. The importance of physical intimacy vacillates throughout a relationship, and may be diminished or rekindled by a superimposed illness. Long-term palliative care providers may see sexual desire and expression ebb and flow between couples throughout the course of care. The patient may view sexual expression as an affirmation of life, a part of being human, a means to maintain role relationships, or the expression of passion in and for life itself. There exists tremendous diversity of cultural, religious, and spiritual beliefs in relation to sexual intimacy and death. Culture often guides interactions between people, and even the mores within sexual interactions. Culturally competent healthcare providers should take into consideration the effect of culture on sexual expression. For example, do both members of the couple possess the same cultural identity? If not, are their identities similar with respect to beliefs about intimacy? What are the couple's health, illness, and sexual beliefs and practices? What are their customs and beliefs about intimacy, illness, and death? Issues such as personal space, eye contact, touch, and permissible topics to discuss with healthcare providers and/or members of the opposite sex may influence one's ability to intercede within the realm of intimate relations. A cultural assessment is vital to determining whether these factors are an issue. Variations in sexual orientation must also be considered within the area of cultural competence. The beliefs, actions, and normative actions of homosexual and bisexual couples are important considerations when providing palliative care to a couple with alternate sexual expression.[5–8]

Sexual Anatomy and Functioning

Sexual health assumes a basic knowledge, understanding, and acceptance of one's sexual anatomy, sexual response, and sexual functioning, as well as freedom from sexual dysfunction and other sexual problems.[1] Physical sexual expression is a basic aspect of human life, seen by many as fundamental to "being human." It is a complex phenomenon that basically comprises the greatest intimacy between two humans. The ability to give and to receive physical love is very important for many individuals, throughout the trajectory of an incurable illness.[9,10] The ability to maintain close sexual relations can be viewed as maintaining an essential part of one's "self." Sexuality can affirm love, relieve stress and anxiety, and distract one from the emotional and physical sequelae of a life-threatening chronic illness. Sexual expression can foster hope and accentuate spirituality. Healthcare providers in all clinical settings where palliative care is provided can be pivotal in facilitating the expression of sexuality in the terminal stages of life. Holistic palliative care throughout the trajectory of an illness should include the promotion of sexual expression and assistance in preventing or minimizing the negative effects of disease progression on a couple's intimacy. Sexual partners' caring can comfortably include sexual expression if both parties are interested and able.

Sexual Healthcare and Safer Sex

As a component of the sexual health model, physical health includes, but is not limited to, practicing safer sex behaviors, knowing one's body, obtaining regular exams, and responding to physical changes with appropriate medical interventions.[1] The promotion or restoration of sexual health begins with a sexual assessment.

Sexual Assessment

Assessment should include the patient as well as his or her partner. Securing permission to include the sexual partner is necessary. Perceived insufficient knowledge on the part of the healthcare provider is often an obstacle to frank sexual discussions.[11,12]

Assessment of sexuality begins with a sexual history, and is then supplemented by data regarding the patient's and partner's physical health as it influences intimacy, psychological sequelae of the chronic illness, sociocultural influences, and possible environmental issues.[13] Sexual health varies from person to person, so it is essential to determine whether the couple is satisfied with their current level of sexual functioning.[14] Celibacy, for example, may have been present in the relationship for years. However, the trajectory of palliative care may have forced celibacy on an otherwise sexually active couple.[15] Determining the couple's need for interventions and assistance in this area is vital to determining appropriate interventions.

Obtaining a sexual history and performing a subsequent sexual assessment can be augmented using several communication techniques—assuring privacy and confidentiality; allowing for ample, uninterrupted time; and maintaining a nonjudgmental attitude. Addressing the topic of sexuality early in the relationship with a palliative care patient legitimizes the issue of intimacy.[16] It delivers the message that this is an appropriate topic for concern within the professional relationship, and is often met with relief on the part of the patient and couple. Often, sexuality concerns are present but unvoiced.[4]

Incorporating several techniques of therapeutic communication enhances the interview. These techniques include asking open-ended questions ("Some people who have an incurable illness are frustrated by their lack of private time with their spouse/sexual partner. How is this experience for you?"); using questions that refer to frequency as opposed to occurrence ("How often do you have intimate relations with your wife/husband/partner?" as opposed to "Do you have intimate relations with your wife/husband/partner?"); and "unloading" the question ("Some couples enjoy oral sex on a regular basis, while others seldom or never have oral sex. How often do you engage in oral sex?"). This last technique legitimizes the activity and allows the patient to feel safe in responding to the question in a variety of ways.[13]

Gender and age may also play a part in the patient's comfort with sexual discussions. An adolescent boy may feel more comfortable discussing sexual concerns with a male healthcare provider, whereas an elder woman may prefer to discuss sexual issues with a woman closer to her own age. Assessment of these factors may include statements like the following: "Many young men have questions about sexuality and the effect their illness may have on sexual functioning. This is something we can discuss or, if you'd be more comfortable, I could have one of the male nurses talk to you about this. Which would you prefer?"[13]

If the sexual history reveals a specific sexual problem, a more in-depth assessment is warranted. This would include the onset and course of the problem, the patient's or couple's thoughts about what caused the problem, any solutions that have been attempted, and potential solutions and their acceptability to the patient/couple. For example, use of a vibrator in the case of male impotence may be entirely acceptable to some couples but abhorrent to others. Determining what is and is not acceptable regarding potential solutions is part of the logical next step in sexual assessment.

Finally, documentation in the patient's chart should reflect the findings of the sexual assessment. Many institutions have a section for sexual assessment embedded within their intake form. This can be completed, and more thorough notes added to the narrative section on the chart. Findings, suggestions for remediation, and desired outcomes should be documented. This will prevent duplication of efforts, enhance communication within the healthcare team, and support continuity of care within the realm of sexual health.

Challenges: Overcoming Barriers to Sexual Health

Challenges to sexual health include previous sexual history, developmental issues, privacy, and physical symptoms or side effects of symptom management.[7] Previous sexual history such as sexual abuse, substance abuse, compulsive sexual behavior, sex work, harassment, and discrimination are critical in any discussion of sexual health. This is particularly true in the context of interventions for cultural and sexual minorities, many of whom are disproportionately affected by these issues.[1] It is not uncommon to see our patients only as they present to us, without full appreciation of their previous life histories.

Developmental Issues

There are a number of developmental issues that may play a part in the patient's ability to maintain intimacy during palliative care.[17] Often, healthcare providers assume sexual abstinence in the elderly and, to some degree, in adolescents and unmarried young adults.[18] However, intimacy may be a vital part of these individuals' lives.[19]

Chronological age may or may not be a determination of sexual activity.[20] For underage patients, parental influence may interfere with the ability to express physical love. Likewise, older adults may be inhibited by perceived societal values and judgments about their sexuality.[19–25] Maintaining an open, nonjudgmental approach to patients of all ages, sexual orientations, and marital status when assessing sexual health may foster trust and facilitate communication.

Privacy

One of the main external challenges to maintaining intimate relations during palliative care is the lack of privacy. In the acute care setting, privacy is often difficult to achieve. However, this obstacle can be removed or minimized by recognizing the need for intimacy and making arrangements to ensure quiet, uninterrupted time for couples. Private rooms are, of course, ideal. However, if this is not possible, arranging for roommates and visitors to leave for periods of time is necessary. A sign could be posted on the door that alerts healthcare providers, staff, and visitors that privacy is required. Finally, many rooms in the acute care setting have windows as opposed to walls, requiring the use of blinds and/or curtains to assure privacy. The nurse should offer such strategies rather than expecting patients to request privacy. Similar issues may arise in the long-term care environment.[23] If privacy is a scarce commodity, assisting couples to maintain desired intimate relations is crucial in providing holistic care. Nurses in long-term care settings can initiate strategies to offer privacy. Such privacy may be more important than in acute care settings, because the stay in long-term care is usually quite extended.[26] In both the acute care and long-term care settings, nurses can play a vital role in setting policy to facilitate the expression of intimacy and the maintenance of sexual health. Home care may present an array of different obstacles for maintaining intimate relations, such as the ongoing presence of a healthcare provider other than the sexual partner. The home setting is often interrupted by professional visits as well as visits from family, friends, and clergy, which may be unplanned or unannounced. The telephone itself may be an unwelcome interruption. Often, when receiving home hospice care, the patient may have been moved from a more private bedroom setting to a more convenient central location, such as a den or family room, to aid caregiving and to enable the patient to maintain an integral role in family life. However, this move does not provide the privacy usually sought for intimate activity. There may not be a door to close; proximity of the patient's bed to the main rooms of the house may inhibit a couple's intimate activities, and they may need to schedule private time together. Necessary steps to maintain sexual relations include scheduling "rest periods" when one will not be disturbed; turning the ringer of the phone off; asking healthcare providers, friends, and clergy to call before visiting; and having family members respect periods of uninterrupted time.

Fatigue

Fatigue may be secondary to many factors. Fatigue may render a patient unable to perform sexually. If fatigue is identified as a factor in the patient's ability to initiate or maintain sexual arousal, several strategies may be suggested to diminish these untoward effects.[27] Minimizing exertion during intimate relations may be necessary. Providing time for rest before and after sexual relations is often a sufficient strategy to overcome the detrimental effects of fatigue. Likewise, avoiding the stress of a heavy meal, alcohol consumption, or extremes in temperature may be helpful. Experimenting with positions that require minimal patient exertion (male-patient, female astride; female-patient, male astride) is often helpful. Finally, timing should be taken into consideration. Sexual activity in the morning upon awakening may be preferable to relations at the end of a long day. Planning for intimate time may replace spontaneity, but this can be a beneficial trade-off.

Pain

Sexual health can be impaired by the presence of pain and by the use of pain medication (especially opiates), which can interfere with sexual arousal.[28] The goal of pain therapy is to alleviate or minimize discomfort; however, attaining that goal may result in an alteration in sexual responsiveness (i.e., libido or erectile function). Temporarily adjusting pain medications, or experimenting with complementary methods of pain management, should be explored. For example, using relaxation techniques and/or romantic music may decrease discomfort through distraction and relaxation, while enhancing sexual interest. Physical sexual activity itself can be viewed as a form of distraction and subsequent relaxation. The couple should be encouraged to explore positions that offer the most comfort. Traditional positions may be abandoned for more comfortable ones, such as sitting in a chair or taking a side-lying position. Pillows can be used to support painful limbs or to maintain certain positions. A warm bath or shower before sexual activity may help pain relief and be seen as preparatory to intimate relations. Massage can be used as both an arousal technique and a therapeutic strategy for minimizing discomfort. Finally, suggesting the exploration of alternate ways of expressing tenderness and sexual gratification may be necessary if the couple's traditional intimacy repertoire is not feasible due to discomfort.

Nausea and Vomiting

Nausea and vomiting are common during the palliative care trajectory and negatively impact sexual health. There are many medications that suppress nausea; however, they may interfere with sexual functioning due to their sedative effects. If the patient complains of sexual difficulties secondary to treatment for nausea and vomiting, assess which antiemetics are prescribed and try another medication and/or use alternate nonpharmacological methods to control nausea and vomiting. As with fatigue, timing may be an important consideration for intimate relations. If the patient/couple notes that nausea is more prevalent during a certain time of the day, planning for intimacy at alternate times may circumvent this problem.[27]

Neutropenia and Thrombocytopenia

Neutropenia and thrombocytopenia, per se, do not necessarily interfere with intimacy, but they do pose some potential problems. Sexual intimacy during neutropenic phases may jeopardize the compromised patient, because severe neutropenia predisposes the patient to infections. Close physical contact may be inadvisable if the sexual partner has a communicable disease, such as an upper respiratory infection or influenza. Specific sexual practices, such as anal intercourse, are prohibited during neutropenic states due to the likelihood of subsequent infection. The absolute neutrophil count, if available, is a good indicator of neutropenic status and associated risk for infection. Patient and partner education about the risks associated with neutropenia is essential.

Thrombocytopenia and the associated risk of bleeding, bruising, or hemorrhage should be considered when counseling a couple about intimacy issues. Again, anal intercourse is contraindicated due to risk for bleeding. Likewise, vigorous genital intercourse may cause vaginal bleeding. Indeed, even forceful or energetic hugging, massage, or kissing may cause bruising or bleeding. Preventative suggestions might include such strategies as gentle lovemaking, with minimal pressure on the thrombocytopenic patient, or having the patient assume the dominant position to control force and pressure.

Dyspnea

Dyspnea is an extremely distressing occurrence in the end-of-life trajectory. Dyspnea, or even the fear of initiating dyspnea, can impair sexual functioning.[29] General strategies can be employed to minimize dyspnea during sexual play. These can include using a waterbed to accentuate physical movements, raising the dyspneic patient's head and shoulders to facilitate oxygenation, using supplementary oxygen and/or inhalers before and during sexual activity, performing pulmonary hygiene measures before intimacy, encouraging slower movements to conserve energy, and modifying sexual activity to allow for enjoyment and respiratory comfort.[30,31]

Neuropathies

Neuropathies can be a result of disease progression or complication of prior treatment. Neuropathies can manifest as pain, paresthesia, and/or weakness. Depending on the location and severity of the neuropathy, sexual functioning can be altered or completely suppressed. Management or diminution of the neuropathy may or may not be feasible. If not, creative ways to evade the negative sequelae of this occurrence are necessary. Such strategies might include creative positioning, use of pillows to support affected body parts, or alternate ways of expressing physical love. The distraction of physical sexual expression may temporarily minimize the perception of the neuropathy.

Mobility and Range of Motion

Mobility issues and compromised range of motion may interfere with sexual expression. Similar to issues related to fatigue, a decrease in mobility can inhibit a couple's customary means of expressing physical love.[32] A compromise in range of motion can result in a similar dilemma. For example, a female patient may no longer be able to position herself in such a way as to allow penile penetration from above due to hip or back restrictions. Likewise, a male patient may have knee or back restrictions that make it impossible for him to be astride his partner. Regardless of the exact nature of the range-of-motion/mobility concern, several suggestions can be offered. Anti-inflammatory medication before sexual activity, experimenting with alternate positions, employing relaxation techniques before sexual play, massage, warm baths, and exploring alternative methods of expressing physical intimacy should be encouraged.[33]

Erectile Dysfunction

Erectile dysfunction can be caused by physiological, psychological, and emotional factors.[34] These factors include vascular, endocrine, and neurological causes; chronic diseases, such as renal failure[35] and diabetes; and iatrogenic factors, such as surgery and medications. Surgical severing of the small nerve branches essential for erection is often a side-effect of radical pelvic surgery, radical prostatectomy, and aortoiliac surgery.[6] Vascular and neurological causes may not be reversible, although endocrine causes may be minimized. For example, the use of estrogen in advanced prostate cancer may be terminated in palliative care, which may result in the return of erectile function. Many medications decrease desire and erectile capacity in men. The most common offenders are antihypertensives, antidepressants, antihistamines, antispasmodics, sedatives or tranquilizers, barbiturates, sex hormone preparations, opioids, and psychoactive drugs.[36] Often, these medications cannot be discontinued to permit the return of erectile function; for those patients, penile implants may be an option.[37]

The uses of sildenafil (Viagra), vardenafil HCl (Levitra), tadalafil (Cialis), and yohimbine (Yohimbine) have not been researched with patients receiving palliative care. These medications are classified as selective enzyme inhibitors. They relax smooth muscle, increase blood flow, and facilitate erection.[38] If a vascular component is part of the underlying erectile dysfunction, the use of one of these medications may correct the problem.[39] Contraindications such as underlying heart disease and other current medications should be taken into consideration.[40] Otherwise, if acceptable to the couple, digital or oral stimulation of the female partner or use of a vibrator can be suggested.[41]

Dyspareunia

Dyspareunia, like erectile dysfunction, can be caused by physiological, psychological, and emotional factors. These factors include vascular, endocrine, and neurological causes as well as iatrogenic factors such as surgery and medications.[42,43] Vascular and neurological causes may not be reversible; endocrine causes may be minimized. For example, the use of estrogen replacement therapy (ERT), vaginal estrogen creams (estrogen replacement is contraindicated for women with hormone receptor-positive tumors), or water-soluble lubricants may be helpful in diminishing vaginal dryness, which can cause painful intercourse. Gynecological surgery and pelvic irradiation may result in physiological changes that prevent comfortable intercourse.[44]

Postirradiation changes, such as vaginal shortening, thickening, and narrowing, may result in severe dyspareunia.[45] For women, as with male patients, many medications decrease desire and function. These drugs include antihypertensives, antidepressants, antihistamines, antispasmodics, sedatives or tranquilizers, barbiturates, sex hormone preparations, opioids, and psychoactive drugs. Often, these medications cannot be discontinued in order to facilitate the return of sexual health. For those patients, digital or oral stimulation of the male partner may be suggested, if acceptable. Additionally, intrathigh and intramammary penetration may be suggested to women who find vaginal intercourse too painful. See Table 1.1 for an overview of dyspareunia management.

Table 1.1 Management of Vaginal Dryness and Dyspareunia

Assess	Comments/Considerations	HCP Management
General History		
Location, onset, intensity of pain	Location may indicate nature of problem (details below)	Give patient the booklet *A-Z Guide for Sexual Health* (mmatzo@ouhsc.edu)
Trend (same or worse over time)	If onset after surgery, may be related to scarring or neuropathic in nature. Pain may increase over time if pelvic muscles involved.	
Resources couple has already utilized Other comorbidities: Sjogren's syndrome, MS, Diabetes, etc.	Diabetics are more prone to yeast infections, decreased lubrication and orgasmic function, and cervical pain.	
General Vaginal Pain		
Bacterial/fungal infections	Diabetics are more prone to yeast infections, decreased lubrication and orgasmic function, and cervical pain. (Patients with MS often experience painful intercourse, decreased lubrication, and decreased sensation).	Treat infection with antibiotics/antifungals.
Assess dryness/atrophy of tissue	If patient unable to localize pain, also consider all causes below. (Patients with MS often experience painful intercourse, decreased lubrication, and decreased sensation).	Adjust medications that may affect lubrication (e.g. antihistamines/anticholinergics). *Educate patient on promoting healthy vaginal environment.* Encourage use of pH-balanced moisturizers, Kegel exercises. Prescribe vaginal dilator and/or vacuum (Eros). As appropriate, give patient information about moisturizer/lubricant, Kegel exercises, dilator, or Eros vacuum. Consider temporary localized estradiol therapy—may be discontinued once lubrication restored with regular stimulation.

(continued)

Table 1.1 (Continued)

Assess	Comments/Considerations	HCP Management
Vulvar Pain		
Assess for vulvar vestibular syndrome by sensory mapping with cotton-tipped applicator	Many women with vestibular pain will also have levator spasm[42]	5% topical lidocaine ointment twice daily by applicator, or overnight by a cotton ball. Tricyclic antidepressants or anticonvulsants for neuropathic component. If levator muscles involved, refer to PT specializing in pelvic floor physiotherapy. Give patient information about pelvic pain and include a list of physical therapists, e.g., http://www.pelvicpainhelp.com/symptoms/levator-ani-syndrome/
Vaginal Vestibule		
Evaluate control of bulbocavernosus muscles		Refer to sexual therapist (or family therapist if relational origin). See Table 1.2, "Management of Psychosocial Issues Contributing to Sexual Problems"
Assess for vaginismus	Primary vaginismus will often have psychosocial components (see negative thoughts/feelings about sex). Secondary vaginismus is reactive to a disease process (i.e., vulvar vestibular syndrome) or relationship issues after a period of successful relations. Levator pain and/or spasm also commonly occur with involuntary contraction of introital muscles.	Patient may benefit from referral for physical therapist specializing in pelvic floor physiotherapy. Give patient information about pelvic pain and include a list of women's health physical therapists.

Mid-Vaginal Pain	
Assess levator muscle tension	Levator spasms can develop as protective response to pelvic pain, and may continue well after original stimulus resolved, continuing the pain cycle.	Refer to physical therapist specializing in pelvic floor physiotherapy. Give patient information about pelvic pain and include a list of women's health physical therapists, e.g., http://www.pelvicpainhelp.com/symptoms/levator-ani-syndrome/

Deep Vaginal Pain		
Assess cervix for neuropathic pain by palpating with cotton-tipped applicator	Pain will be focal, often elicited by palpitation of only one quadrant of cervix.	5% topical lidocaine ointment twice daily by applicator, or overnight by a cotton ball
Rectovaginal exam	Pain can be related to scarring from hysterectomy, repeated trauma, etc.	Tricyclic antidepressants or anticonvulsants for neuropathic component of pain.

Other Causes		
Bladder disease	GI illnesses such as Crohn's disease, irritable bowel	Suspected GI/GU causes: refer to GI/GU specialist
Gastrointestinal illnesses	syndrome can cause visceral hyperalgia	Musculoskeletal pain: Give patient information about
Adnexal pathology	Areas of abdominal point tenderness should be	pelvic pain and include a list of women's health physical
Sensitivity of abdominal wall	evaluated with/without patient raising head off table	therapists, e.g., http://www.pelvicpainhelp.com/symptoms/
Pelvic floor or hip muscle pain	(rectus abdominus flexion). If equal or increased	levator-ani-syndrome/
Other inflammatory or visceral disorders	with abdominal flexion, then myofascial structures	
Postoperative (especially some pelvic support surgeries)	of abdominal wall may be involved in pain generation (Steege & Zolnoun, 2009).	

Psychosocial Factors		
Relationship issues	Anxiety is an independent predictor of dyspareunia,	See Table 1.2, "Management of Psychosocial Issues
Depression, fear, or stress	aside from structural factors.	Contributing to Sexual Problems," for specific referrals.
Past abuse	Vaginismus is often attributed to difficulties with upbringing or discomfort with sexuality in general (Steege & Zolnoun, 2009)	

Anxiety and Depression

Anxiety and depression related to the incurable and terminal aspects of the disease may interfere with sexual desire and response.[46] Both anxiety and depression have profound effects on sexual functioning. Decreases in sexual desire, libido, and activity are common sequelae of these affective disorders. However, some interventions, especially pharmacological management, can further compromise sexual functioning.

A thorough assessment of the patient's psychological state and an evaluation of the medications currently prescribed for this condition may reveal the source of the problem. Anxiolytics and antidepressants are often prescribed for these conditions and have the potential for interfering with sexual functioning. Patients may choose symptom management and sacrifice sexual function. However, relaxation techniques, imagery, and biofeedback may lower anxiety to a tolerable level. Additionally, the release of sexual tension may itself resolve anxiety.

If desire is maintained and function alone is compromised for male patients, the couple may explore alternate ways of pleasing each other. For female patients, use of water-soluble lubricants can offset the interference with arousal, if interest remains intact. Open communication between the partners and with the healthcare provider allows for frank discussions and the presentation of possible alternatives to expressing physical affection (Table 1.2).

Body Image

In a culture with so many sexual images focused on a type of physical beauty unattainable for many, body image is an important aspect of sexual health. Challenging one, narrow standard of beauty and encouraging self-acceptance is relevant to all populations, and should be carried out in a culturally sensitive manner.[1] An incurable illness and concomitant end-of-life care can alter one's physical appearance. Additionally, past treatments for disease often irrevocably alter body appearance and function. Issues such as alopecia, weight loss, cachexia, the presence of a stoma, or amputation of a body part, to name a few, can result in feelings of sexual inadequacy and/or disinterest (Table 1.3).[47,48]

End-of-life care can focus on the identification and remediation of issues related to body image changes. Although an altered appearance may be permanent, counseling and behavior modification, as well as specific suggestions to minimize or mask these appearances, can improve body image to a level compatible with positive sexual health. The use of a wig, scarf, or headbands can mask alopecia. Some patients, rather than try to conceal hair loss, choose to emphasize it by shaving their heads. Weight loss and cachexia can be masked through clothing and the creative use of padding.

The presence of an ostomy can significantly alter body image and negatively affect sexual functioning.[60,61] Specific interventions for minimizing the effect that the presence of an ostomy has on sexual functioning depend, in

Table 1.2 Management of Psychosocial Issues Contributing to Sexual Problems

Assess	Comments/Considerations	HCP Management
Body Image (NCCN Guideline for Distress: DIS-6; MS-8,9)*		
Fertility	Premenopausal women	Encourage patient to attend an infertility support group.
		Give patient information about fertility, e.g., http://www.fertilehope.org/; http://www.cancer.org/treatment/treatmentsandsideeffects/ physicalsideeffects/fertilityandcancer whataremyoptions/fertility-and-cancer-toc;
Loss of Womanhood	Express concern of self-image	Refer for counseling
Hair loss		Encourage patient to attend a support group.
Scars		
Colostomy		Encourage patient to attend an ostomy support group.
		Give patient the booklet *Intimacy After Ostomy Surgery* (http://www.ostomy.org/ostomy_info/pubs/uoaa_sexuality_en.pdf) with the list of supports groups attached.
Emotional (NCCN Guideline for Distress: DIS-6; MS-2,8,9)*		
Anxiety	Symptoms: Loss of appetite, sleep, or concentration;	Prescribe medications (anxiolytic, antidepressant).
Fear	Preoccupied with thoughts of illness/death;	Suggest integrative therapies—i.e., yoga, exercise, mediation, walking club, laughter club, etc.
Depression	Sadness at loss of health; Anger, feeling out of control.	Encourage to attend a support group.
	If managing symptoms with medication, consider impact on sexual function.	Refer for counseling
Spiritual (NCCN Guideline for Distress: DIS-19,20; MS-9)*		
Spiritual conflict	Most cancer patients have spiritual needs, but only a slight	Refer to chaplain
Grief/guilt	majority felt it was appropriate to ask about these needs.	
Hopelessness	Cancer patients can experience an existential crisis.	

(continued)

Table 1.2 (Continued)

Practical Concerns *(NCCN Guideline for Distress: DIS-18; MS-9*)*

Finances Housing Transportation Isolation	Question if the patient's concrete needs are met. Ask the patient about her living/support situation	Refer to social work services
Cultural/language issues	Does the patient have a language barrier?	Ask patient to bring a translator to clinic visits or provide one if needed. Spanish-speaking cancer support groups are available throughout the country.

Psychosocial *(NCCN Guideline for Distress: DIS-6; MS-3*)*

Adjustment to illness Family conflicts Social isolation	Functional changes affecting quality of life issues. Help with coping or communication skills or with difficulties in decision-making	Refer to social work services
Domestic abuse/neglect	Signs of possible abuse or neglect:** Failure to keep appointments, secrecy, discomfort when interviewed about relationship, partner will not leave patient alone with medical staff, unexplained/multiple injuries, chronic pain without apparent etiology, high number of STIs, pregnancies, miscarriages, and abortions.	
Advanced directives End-of-life issues		

Relationships *(NCCN Guideline for Distress: DIS-19; MS-3,9)**

Partner	Communication with partner about sexual health or needs	Refer to AASECT sexual therapist Give patient information about sexual therapists in your area Refer for counseling Give patient information about marriage counseling.
Family	Children of patients with difficulties coping	Give patient information on support groups for children in your area

* Comprehensive Cancer Network (NCCN) Clinical Practice Guidelines in Oncology. Distress Management. www.nccn.org. 2013; V.2.2013.

** National Consensus Guidelines on Identifying and Responding to Domestic Violence Victimization in Health Care Setting. *The Family Violence Prevention Fund* http://www.endabuse.org/userfiles/file/Consensus.pdf; 2004;Appendix G "Indicators of Abuse"(February 2004):page 43.

Table 1.3 Management of Loss of Libido

Assess	Comments/Considerations	HCP Management
Psychosocial Factors[1,2]		
Relationship issues Depression, fear, or stress Past abuse Poor body image	Referral to mental health professional or social services (See Table 1.2, "Management of Psychosocial Issues Contributing to Sexual Problems")	
Medications That Can Impact Desire		

Antidepressants (especially SSRIs) Antihypertensives/ cardiovascular
H2 blockers
	Some substitutions may be possible within same drug class which have less of an impact on sexual functioning	For Antidepressants[3-8]
		1. Adjust current antidepressant dosing
		2. Alter timing of dose (so decreased serum levels when most likely to be sexually active)
		3. 2-day "drug holidays" (effective for sertraline and paroxitine)
		4. Substitution with another medication:
		  a. Minimal to no sexual dysfunction: bupropion, maritazapine
		  b. Low risk of sexual dysfunction: fluvoxamine, citalopram, venlafaxine

Unfavorable Experiences due to Pain		
See Table 1.2, "Management of Psychosocial Issues Contributing to Sexual Problems"		**Cancer-Related Pain:** NCCN Clinical Guideline: Adult Cancer Pain
	Vaginismus can result from dyspareunia, contributing to pain cycle and fear of sexual intimacy	**Dyspareunia:** See Table 1.1, "Management of Vaginal Dryness and Dyspareunia." **Vaginismus:** may need referral to mental health professional, especially if patient experienced prolonged dyspareunia or contributing psychosocial factors.[9]

(continued)

Table 1.3 (Continued)

Assess	Comments/Considerations	HCP Management
Fatigue (NCCN Clinical Guideline: Cancer Treatment Related Fatigue: MS 8–13)[10]		
Cancer-related fatigue is a distressing persistent, subjective sense of physical, emotional, and/or cognitive tiredness or exhaustion related to cancer or cancer treatment that is not proportional to recent activity and interferes with usual functioning.	Fatigue can be a result of inactivity. Some patients may benefit by gradually increasing their daily exercise. Patients should be counseled about coping and educated on how to deal with anxiety and depression, which are commonly associated with fatigue. Poor nutrition may contribute to fatigue. Consider psychostimulants to combat fatigue.	**Nonpharmacologic interventions** (MS–8 – M-11) 1. Activity enhancement and physically based therapies: Give the patient the hand-out "Physical Activity and the Cancer Patient." 2. Psychosocial interventions: Refer to counselor 3. Nutritional consultation: Refer active patients (in treatment) to a nutritionist. Include with the referral a patient assessment form that the patient can bring with her on her first visit with the dietician. **Pharmacologic interventions** (M-12 – M-13) 1. Amphetamine psychostimulant Methylphenidate *Only beneficial in severe fatigue or and/or advanced disease* 2. Nonamphetamine psychostimulant Modfinil 3. For anemia Erythropoietin
Hormones		
Hormone Levels Cortisol Free testosterone (or FTI/FAI)	High cortisol levels can compete with androgenic hormones. Decreased androgen levels with surgical menopause can be significant factor in HSDD. Supplementation is controversial, but increasing evidence supports safety and efficacy of transdermal medications. Consider supplementation if free testosterone levels for women: Under 50: <25 ng/dL or 1.5 pg/mL Over 50: <20 ng/dL or <1.0 ng/mL	**High cortisol levels:** encourage stress-reducing activities. Consider mental health referral for patients experiencing psychosocial situations contributing to stress (See Table 1.2. "Management of Psychosocial Issues Contributing to Sexual Problems"). **Low Testosterone:** No FDA-approved testosterone products for treating HSDD in women, but numerous preparations are commonly prescribed off-label.[11] Transdermal matrix (Intrinsa) shown to be effective at 150–300 mcg/d, with no increase in BrCa Risk. Monitor serum FT for therapeutic effectiveness.

Please see References 49 to 59 for further information.

part, on the particular type of ostomy. Some patients are continent, while others need an appliance attached at all times.

If the patient has a continent ostomy, timing sexual activity can allow for removal of the appliance and covering the stoma. If the ostomy appliance cannot be safely removed, the patient should be taught to empty the appliance before intimate relations and to use a cover or body stocking to conceal the appliance. Alternate positions may also be considered, and in the event of a leak, sexual activity can continue in the shower. The United Ostomy Association (http://www.uoa.org) publishes four patient information booklets on sexuality and the ostomate.

Masturbation and Fantasy

The topics of masturbation and fantasy are saddled with a myriad of historical myths associated with sin, illness, and immaturity that would need to be confronted in order to normalize masturbation. Encouraging masturbation as a normal adjunct to partnered sex can decrease the pressures on people to engage in penetrative sex with their partners more frequently than they have desire and arousal for.[1]

Some patients may view sexual expression as an essential aspect of their being, while others may see it as ancillary or unimportant. Some may have an established sexual partner; some may lose a partner through separation, divorce, or death; others may begin a relationship during the course of their illness trajectory. Some patients may have several sexual partners; some couples may be gay or lesbian; others, without a sexual partner, may gain pleasure by erotic thoughts and masturbation. All of these scenarios are within the realm of the palliative care provider's patient base. Understanding the various forms of sexual expression and pleasure is paramount in providing comprehensive care.

Intimacy and Relationships

Intimacy is a universal need that people try to meet through their relationships.[1] A sexual partner's interest and ability to maintain sexual relations throughout the palliative care trajectory can also be affected by many variables. Sexual expression may be impeded by the partner's mood state (anxiety, depression, grief, or guilt), exhaustion from caregiving and assuming multiple family roles, and misconceptions about sexual appropriateness during palliative care. Anxiety and depression have profound effects on sexual functioning. Decreases in libido and sexual activity can result from depressive and anxious states.[62,63]

A partner may feel that the patient is "too ill" to engage in sexual activity. In turn, the partner may feel remorse or guilt for even thinking about their loved one in a sexual capacity during this time. Partners may fear that they may injure their loved one during sexual activity due to the loved one's perceived or actual weakened state or appearance. The partner may have difficulty adjusting to the altered physical appearance of the patient (cachexia, alopecia, stomatitis, pallor, amputation, etc.). The role of caregiver may seem incompatible with that of sexual partner.

As the ill partner's health deteriorates, the well partner may assume caretaking roles that may seem incompatible with those of a lover. The myriad of responsibilities sequentially assumed by the well partner may leave him or her exhausted, which can interfere with sexual health and impede sexual performance. The partner may harbor misconceptions about sexual relations with a terminally ill partner, including diminishing the patient's waning energy reserves or causing the illness to progress more rapidly.

Spirituality and Values

Sexual health assumes congruence between one's ethical, spiritual, and moral beliefs and one's sexual behaviors and values. In this context, spirituality may or may not include identification with formal religions, but it addresses moral and ethical concerns. Exposure to multiple cultural traditions (e.g., Native American storytelling, African American church activism, etc.) is important, especially in those traditions that have a positive and life-affirming view of sexuality.[1]

Individual, family, and cultural factors influence the development of healthy sexuality in adolescents. One factor that is less often considered, but may play a role, is religion/spirituality. Attitudes or beliefs about having sex before marriage, decisions about the timing of coital debut, or contraceptive practices may be shaped by their religious/spiritual belief system or the cultural/religious context in which they were raised.[64] These values may influence the decisions that an adolescent with a life-limiting disease may make regarding sexual experiences that they choose to engage in before they die.

Interventions

The specific sexual needs and concerns of the patient and couple determine the approach and type of intervention. The intervention can address current needs or focus on potential future needs in the form of anticipatory guidance. False assumptions about intimacy during palliative care can be addressed, and anticipatory guidance regarding what to expect as a result of advancing disease and palliative treatment is included in this discussion.

Specific suggestions should go beyond limited information, and be explicit, to help the patient and their partner attain a mutually stated goal. Specific suggestions usually pertain to communication, symptom management, and alternate physical expression. Open communication between the couple and their healthcare practitioner regarding sexual health is essential for successful symptom management. Candid discussions regarding their emotional responses to this phase of their relationship, their fears and concerns, and their hopes and desires are included in these interactions.

Symptom management is essential to optimizing sexual expression. Alternate expressions of physical intimacy may be necessary if sexual disruption is due to organic changes. If intercourse is difficult, painful, or impossible, the couple may be counseled regarding how to expand their sexual repertoire. A thorough discussion of the couple's values, attitudes, and preferences should be done before suggesting alternatives. Using language that is understandable to the patient/partner is essential. However, the use of slang or street language may be uncomfortable to the healthcare practitioner—defining terms early in the discussion will alleviate this potential problem.

There are many ways of giving and receiving sexual pleasure; genital intercourse is only one way of expressing physical love. The nurse can encourage the couple to expand their sexual expression to include hugging, massage, fondling, caressing, cuddling, kissing, handholding, and masturbation, either mutually or singularly. Sexual gratification may be derived from manual, oral, and digital stimulation. Intrathigh, anal, and intramammary intercourse are also options if the female partner is unable to continue vaginal penetration.

Summary

Incurable illness and end-of-life care may result in compromising a couple's intimacy. To prevent or minimize this, healthcare practitioners should assume a leading role in the assessment and remediation of potential or identified alterations in sexual functioning. Not all couples will be concerned about their sexual health at this point of their life together. However, if sexual health is desired, all attempts should be made to facilitate this important aspect of life. People may find that being physically close to the one they love is life affirming and comforting.

As patients draw close to the end of life, their needs, hopes, and concerns remain intact as in any other stage of their life. Assessment of sexual health should occur for all patients to determine whether these needs and hopes include maintenance of their sexual health. The healthcare practitioner's offer of information and support can make a significant difference in a couple's ability to adjust to the changes in sexual health during end-of-life care.

References

1. Robinson BBE, Bockting WO, Simon Rosser BR, Miner M, Coleman E. The sexual health model: application of a sexological approach to HIV prevention. Health Educ Res. 2002;17(1):43–57.

2. Institute of Medicine. Cancer Care for the Whole Patient: Meeting Psychosocial Health Needs. Washington, DC: National Academies Press; 2007.

3. Young P. Caring for the whole patient: the Institute of Medicine proposes a new standard of care. Community Oncol. 2007;4(12):748–751.

4. Krychman ML, Pereira L, Carter J, Amsterdam A. Sexual oncology: sexual health issues in women with cancer. Oncology. 2006;71(1–2):18–25.

5. Alfano CM, Rowland JH. Recovery issues in cancer survivorship: a new challenge for supportive care. Cancer J. 2006;12(5):432–443.

6. Galbraith ME, Crighton F. Alterations of sexual function in men with cancer. Semin Oncol Nurs. 2008;24(2):102–114.

7. Shell JA. Sexual issues in the palliative care population. Semin Oncol Nurs. 2008;24(2):131–134.

8. Dibble SL, Eliason MJ, Christiansen MAD. Chronic illness care for lesbian, gay, and bisexual individuals. Nurs Clin North Am. 2007;42(4):655–674.

9. Hordern AJ, Currow DC. A patient-centered approach to sexuality in the face of life-limiting illness. Med J Aust. 2003;179(6 Suppl):S8–11.

10. Rice A. Sexuality in cancer and palliative care 1: Effects of disease and treatment. Int J Palliat Nurs. 2000;6(8):392–397.

11. Krebs LU. Sexual assessment: research and clinical. Nurs Clin North Am. 2007;42(4):515–529.

12. Hordern A, Street A. Communicating about patient sexuality and intimacy after cancer: mismatched expectations and unmet needs. Med J Aust. 2007;186(5):224–227.

13. Sadovsky R, Nusbaum M. Sexual health inquiry and support is a primary care priority. J Sex Med. 2006;3(1):3–11.

14. Higgins A, Barker P, Begley CM. Sexuality: the challenge to espoused holistic care. Int J Nurs Pract. 2006;12(6):345–351.

15. Sanders S, Pedro LW, Bantum EO, Galbraith ME. Couples surviving prostate cancer: long-term intimacy needs and concerns following treatment. Clin J Oncol Nurs. 2006;(4):503–508

16. Huber C, Ramnarace T, McCaffrey R. Sexuality and intimacy issues facing women with breast cancer. Oncol Nurs Forum. 2006;33(6):1163–1167.

17. Stausmire JM. Sexuality at the end of life. Am J Hosp Palliat Care. 2004;21(1):33–39.

18. Stroberg P, Hedelin H, Bergstrom AB. Is sex only for the healthy and wealthy? J Sex Med. 2007;4(1):176–182.

19. Hurd Clarke L. Older women and sexuality: experiences in marital relationships across the life course. Can J Aging. 2006;25(2):129–140.

20. Lindau ST, Schumm LP, Laumann EO, Levinson W, O'Muircheartaigh CA, Waite LJ. A study of sexuality and health among older adults in the United States. N Engl J Med. 2007;357:762–774.

21. Lesser J, Hughes S, Kumar S. Sexual dysfunction in the older woman: complex medical, psychiatric illnesses should be considered in evaluation and management. Psychiatric Consultant. 2005;60(8):18–22.

22. Loehr J, Verma S, Seguin V. Issues of sexuality in older women. J Women's Health. 1997;6(4):451–457.

23. Malatesta VJ. Sexual problems, women and aging: an overview. J Women Aging. 2007;19(1–2):139–54.

24. Scott LD. Sexuality and older women: exploring issues while promoting health. AWHONN Lifelines 2002;6(6):520–525.

25. Robinson JG, Molzahn AE. Sexuality and quality of life. J Gerontol Nurs. 2007;33(3):19–29.

26. Everett B, Everett B. Supporting sexual activity in long-term care. Nurs Ethics. 2008;15(1):87–96.

27. Stead ML. Sexual function after treatment for gynecological malignancy. Curr Opin Oncol. 2004;16:492–495.

28. Abs R, Verhelst J, Maeyaert J, et al. Endocrine consequences of long-term intrathecal administration of opioids. J Clin Endocrinol Metab. 2000;85(6):2215–2222.

29. Vincent EE, Singh SJ. Review article: addressing the sexual health of patients with COPD: the needs of the patient and implications for health care professionals. Chron Respir Dis. 2007;4(2):111–115.

30. Hardin S. Cardiac disease and sexuality: implications for research and practice. Nurs Clin North Am. 2007;42(4):593–603.

31. Goodell TT. Sexuality in chronic lung disease. Nurs Clin North Am. 2007;42(4):631–638.

32. Newman AM. Arthritis and sexuality. Nurs Clin North Am. 2007;42(4):621–630.

33. Kautz DD. Hope for love: practical advice for intimacy and sex after stroke . . . including commentary by Secrest J. Rehabil Nurs. 2007;32(3):95–103.

34. Resendes LA, McCorkle R. Spousal responses to prostate cancer: an integrative review. Informa Healthc. 2006;24:192–198.

35. Katz A. What have my kidneys got to do with my sex life?: the impact of late-stage chronic kidney disease on sexual function. Am J Nurs. 2006;106(9):81–83.

36. Karadeniz T, Topsakal M, Aydogmus A, et al. Erectile dysfunction under age 40: etiology and role of contributing factors. ScientificWorldJournal. 2004;4(Suppl 1):171–174.

37. Mulcahy JJ, Wilson SK. Current use of penile implants in erectile dysfunction. Curr Urol Rep. 2006;7(6):485–489.

38. Ali ST. Effectiveness of sildenafil citrate (Viagra) and tadalafil (Cialis) on sexual responses in Saudi men with erectile dysfunction in routine clinical practice. Pak J Pharm Sci. 2008;21(3):275–281.

39. Hartmann U, Burkart M. Erectile dysfunctions in patient–physician communication: optimized strategies for addressing sexual issues and the benefit of using a patient questionnaire. J Sex Med. 2007;4(1):38–46.

40. Ezzell A, Baum N. When Viagra doesn't work: treating erectile dysfunction. Diabetes Self-Management. 2008;25(2):29–30.

41. Bruner DW, Calvano T. The sexual impact of cancer and cancer treatments in men. Nurs Clin North Am. 2007;42(4):555–580.

42. Steege JF, Zolnoun DA. Evaluation and treatment of dyspareunia. Obstet Gynecol. 2009;113(5):1124–1136.

43. Stead ML. Sexual function after treatment for gynecological malignancy. Curr Opin Oncol. 2004;16(5):492–495.

44. Carmack Taylor CL, Basen-Engquist K, Shinn EH, et al. Predictors of sexual functioning in ovarian cancer patients. J Clin Oncol. 2004;22(5):881–889.

45. Yamamoto R, Okamoto K, Ebina Y, Shirato H, Sakuragi N, Fujimoto S. Prevention of vaginal shortening following radical hysterectomy. BJOG. 2000;107(7):841–845.

46. Brandberg Y, Sandelin K, Erikson S, et al. Psychological reactions, quality of life, and body image after bilateral prophylactic mastectomy in women at

high risk for breast cancer: a prospective 1-year follow-up study [see comment]. J Clin Oncol. 2008;26(24):3943–3949.

47. Alfano CM, Rowland JH. Recovery issues in cancer survivorship: a new challenge for supportive care. Cancer J. 2006;12(5):432–443.

48. Hinsley R, Hughes R. "The reflections you get": an exploration of body image and cachexia. Int J Palliat Nurs. 2007;13(2):84–89.

49. DeRogatis LR, Graziottin A, Bitzer J, Schmitt S, Koochaki PE, Rodenberg C. Clinically relevant changes in sexual desire, satisfying sexual activity and personal distress as measured by the profile of female sexual function, sexual activity log, and personal distress scale in postmenopausal women with hypoactive sexual desire disorder. J Sex Med. 2009;6(1):175–183.

50. Wylie KR. Sexuality and the menopause. J Br Menopause Soc. 2006;12(4):149–152.

51. Feldhaus-Dahir M. Testosterone for the treatment of hypoactive sexual desire disorder: part II. Urol Nurs. 2009;29(5):386–389, 378.

52. Kanaly KA, Berman JR. Sexual side effects of SSRI medications: potential treatment strategies for SSRI-induced female sexual dysfunction. Curr Womens Health Rep. 2002;2(6):409–416.

53. Kotz K, Alexander JL, Dennerstein L. Estrogen and androgen hormone therapy and well-being in surgically postmenopausal women. J Womens Health (Larchmt). 2006;15(8):898–908.

54. Labbate LA, Grimes J, Hines A, Oleshansky MA, Arana GW. Sexual dysfunction induced by serotonin reuptake antidepressants. J Sex Marital Ther. 1998;24(1):3–12.

55. Montgomery SA, Baldwin DS, Riley A. Antidepressant medications: a review of the evidence for drug-induced sexual dysfunction. J Affect Disord. 2002;69(1–3):119–140.

56. Wierman ME, Basson R, Davis SR, et al. Androgen therapy in women: an Endocrine Society Clinical Practice guideline. J Clin Endocrinol Metab. 2006;91(10):3697–3710.

57. Boardman LA, Stockdale CK. Sexual pain. Clin Obstet Gynecol. 2009;52(4):682–690.

58. National Comprehensive Cancer Network (NCCN) Clinical Practice Guidelines in Oncology (NCCN GuidelinesTM) Version 1.2011. Cancer-Related Fatigue: Interventions for Active Treatment (M-8 – M-13). http://www.nccn.org/index.asp.

59. Amato P, Buster JE. Diagnosis and treatment of hypoactive sexual desire disorder. Clin Obstet Gynecol. 2009;52(4):666–674.

60. Penson RT, Gallagher J, Gioiella ME, et al. Sexuality and cancer: conversation comfort zone. Oncologist. 2000;5(4):336–344.

61. Kilic E, Taycan O, Belli AK, et al. [The effect of permanent ostomy on body image, self-esteem, marital adjustment, and sexual functioning]. Turk Psikiyatri Dergisi. 2007;18(4):302–310.

62. Barton-Burke M, Gustason CJ. Sexuality in women with cancer. Nurs Clin North Am. 2007;42(4):531–554.

63. Stead ML, Brown JM, Fallowfield L, Selby P. Communication about sexual problems and sexual concerns in ovarian cancer: a qualitative study. West J Med. 2002;176(1):18–19.

64. Cotton S, Berry D. Religiosity, spirituality, and adolescent sexuality. Adolesc Med State Art Rev. 2007;18(3):471–483.

Chapter 2

Bereavement

Inge B. Corless

This chapter emphasizes grief and loss as universal experiences occurring across the life span. Bereavement takes many forms and is influenced by culture, religious practice, nature of the relationship with the deceased, age of the deceased, and manner of death. In this chapter, terms are defined, types of grief described, grief responses reviewed, and interventions suggested. Grief work involves learning to live with the loss and to incorporate the loss into life moving forward.

> ### Key Points
> - As illness advances patients and families face multiple losses.
> - These losses involve physical and mental health, roles, activities, and relationships.
> - Distinguishing normal grief from pathological, complicated, or prolonged grief allows for appropriate interventions.
> - Nurses and other healthcare providers also experience loss.
> - Grief work involves learning to live with the loss.

Case Study: Young Woman With Lengthy Illness

A young woman, a wife and mother, died after a lengthy illness. She had a 2-year illness-free period that was punctuated by metastases to liver and lung. That is not the important part of her story, although it accounts for her demise. The important part of her story is how beloved she was not only by her immediate and extended family but also by the community of those she had met throughout her life and the community in which she lived. The vivid grief expressed by those in attendance at her funeral is in sharp contrast to the more restrained expression of grief typical at white Anglo-Saxon funerals. Not that all in attendance were Caucasian—the mourners at this funeral represented multiple ethnic groups. Those who were most expressive in their grief were those who, culturally, would have been expected to have a stiff upper lip. Would such a response have occurred had the deceased lived her four score years and ten? How do we account for this response to bereavement?

Definitions

Bereavement is the state of loss resulting from death. Bereavement includes grief and mourning—the inner and outward reactions of the survivor. Bereavement is the period where the survivor feels the pain of the loss, mourns, grieves, and adjusts to a world without the physical, psychological, and social presence of the deceased.

Loss is a generic term that signifies absence of an object, position, ability, or attribute. More recently it has also been applied to the death of an animal or person. Patients, family members, and survivors all experience loss. Loss may occur before the actual death, as the patient and significant others anticipate and experience loss of health, changes in relationships and roles, and loss of life (anticipatory grief). After a death, the survivor experiences the loss of the loved one. Most losses trigger mourning and grief and accompanying feelings, behaviors, and reactions to the loss. A theory of ambiguous loss has been used to discuss the situation of foster children whose caregivers may be physically present but psychologically absent, physically absent but psychologically present, or in transient relationships.[1] Mourning and grief under these circumstances may not receive the recognition that is warranted.

The attributes of loss can be formulated as follows:

1. Loss signifies the absence of a relationship or possession.
2. Each loss is valued differently and ranges from little or no value to great value.
3. The meaning of the loss is determined primarily by the individual sustaining it.

Mourning is the outward, social expression of a loss. Kagawa-Singer describes it as "the social customs and cultural practices that follow a death." [2(p1752)] This definition highlights the external manifestations of the process of separation from the deceased and the ultimate reintegration of the bereaved into the family and, to varying degrees, society. How one outwardly expresses a loss may be dictated by cultural norms, customs, and practices including rituals and traditions. Some cultures may be very emotional and verbal in their expressions of loss, some may show little reaction to loss, others may wail or cry loudly, and some may appear stoic and businesslike. Religious and cultural beliefs may also dictate how long one mourns and how the survivor "should" act during the bereavement period. In addition, outward expression of loss may be influenced by the individual's personality and life experiences. Durkheim stated that "mourning is not a natural movement of private feelings wounded by a cruel loss; it is a duty imposed by the group." [3(p443)] This duty is participation in the customary rituals appropriate to membership in a given group. These rituals and behaviors acknowledge that a loss has occurred for the individual and the group, and that the individual and the group are adjusting their relationships so as to move forward without the presence of the deceased individual.

DeSpelder and Strickland highlighted an important distinction pertinent to mourning. They stated, "The term mourning refers not so much to the reaction to loss but rather to the process by which a bereaved person integrates the loss into his ongoing life."[4(p336)] They continue, "the process is determined at least partly by social and cultural norms for expressing grief."[4(p336)] An outward acknowledgment of loss consists of participation in various death and bereavement rituals. These vary by religious and cultural traditions as well as by personal preferences. For example, In South Africa, a Zulu wife is expected to engage in mourning (ukuzila) for 1 year as a sign of respect.[5]

Whereas ancestor worship is important to varying degrees in Asia, Latin cultures believe in the relationship between life and death, a relationship reflected in practices such as the tradition of bringing food to the cemetery and remaining there all night for the Day of the Dead. "These practices have many functions, including signifying respect for the deceased and providing a mechanism for the expression of feelings by the bereaved. A similar relationship is observed in Africa, where "the living and the dead together constitute the social world."[6(p341)]

Mourning is also expressed in the symbolism entailed in funerals and burials. Burial grounds contain the expressions of what was considered appropriate in each time period for the memorialization of the deceased. These memorials may be above or below ground, in cemeteries or memorial parks, as part of individual graves or mausoleums, or various permutations. The availability of space for burials influences the manner in which burials and memorials are constructed. Various reasons for the visit to cemeteries by mourners include to fulfill obligations, to help achieve independence from the deceased, and to seek solace.[7(p408)]

Grief can be defined as "a reaction to loss—we can experience grief obviously when someone we're attached to dies, but we can also experience it when we lose any significant form of attachment."[8]

The Process of Bereavement

The process and meaning of bereavement varies depending on a number of factors, including age, gender, ethnicity, cultural background, education, and socioeconomic status. For African American widows, storytelling was the means by which the bereavement experience was described.[9] The themes identified in a study of these widows included awareness of death, caregiving, getting through, moving on, changing feelings, and financial security. These themes illustrate many concerns of bereavement.

The impact of grief affects the physical and mental health of the bereaved. An increase in mortality from a variety of causes for the bereaved has been found, including changes in personal habits and social activities and psychological distress; psychological distress can take the form of grief or depression.[10] The distinction between grief and depression in the bereaved is an important one.[11] Middleton and associates[12(p451)] concluded, "The bereaved can experience considerable pain and yet be coping adaptively, and they can fulfill many depressive criteria yet at the same time be experiencing phenomena that are not depressive in nature." Even in individuals with a history of "sadness or irritability" before bereavement, although they may have more intense expressions of grief, the rate of recovery is the same as for those without such a history.[13] Subsyndromal symptomatic depressions are "frequently seen complications of bereavement that may be chronic and often are associated with substantial morbidity."[14(p35)]

Rubin and Schecter conceptualized bereavement-related grief into the two-track model of bereavement as a means of understanding and addressing the bereavement process and its outcome.

Track 1 addresses biopsychological functioning and is concerned with two questions: "Where are the difficulties in biopsychological functioning?" and "Where are the strengths and growth manifest?"[15]

Track 2 examines the relationship to the deceased and focuses on two questions: "What is the state of the desire to reconnect with the deceased affectively and cognitively?" and "What is the nature of the ongoing relationship to the deceased? Is the death story integrated?"[15]

In essence, bereavement involves adjusting to a world without the physical, psychological, and social presence of the deceased. Prebereavement mental distress such as depression and anxiety, as well as a high level of perceived burden with lack of support, have been found to be predictive of a poor bereavement outcome.[16,17] Bereavement becomes complicated when adjustment is impeded, as in posttraumatic stress disorder. Whether such bereavement occurs as a result of vehicular accident, war, or natural disaster, the suddenness or overwhelming nature of the event dislodges the sense that all is well with the world. The sense of disequilibrium is amplified when bereavement is the result of suicide. Such a death is accompanied by an overwhelming sense of guilt and the sense of abandonment and rejection.[18] Even in instances in which an elective medical procedure such as abortion occurs, the emotional response may not become evident until many years later.

Death before its time, as in children and young and middle-aged adults, not only affects the bereaved directly but also affects the social roles of the survivors that require readjustment. The issues occasioned by the death of a child with intellectual disabilities have much in common with disenfranchised grief.[19] Studies have underscored the need for postbereavement support in such cases.[19,20] Disenfranchised grief is compounded by stigma for children with a father on death row, who must contend first with the loss of having an incarcerated parent and then with his death by execution.[21]

The hesitancy of children to exhibit their own sadness so as not to upset their parents requires that professionals encourage parents to give their children permission to be sad when that is how they feel. In a study that sought to identify those factors that helped or hindered adolescent sibling bereavement, a youngster stated:

> "What helped me the most was my mother, who was totally honest with me from the time Sarah got sick through her death. My mother took the time to listen to how I felt as well as understand and hug me."[22]

Adolescents whose parents died of cancer have been noted to be more likely to engage in self-injury with a range in prevalence of from 6% to 40%.[23] The importance of support for children and adolescents cannot be overstated.

Situations where individuals are expected to "get on with it" may pose difficulties for those who are bereaved.[24] Personality correlates were found to influence bereavement narratives.[25] Cognitive processing and finding meaning can be helpful to a variety of individuals. Older persons have been noted to be more reluctant to express their feelings.[26] Routine bereavement care can be helpful in identifying people at risk for complicated grieving. For individuals who would like to join a support group but are unable to do so for a variety of reasons of time, distance, or responsibilities, an Internet support group may be an option.[27] Palliative care teams play an important role in identifying caregivers at risk for bereavement difficulties so that early intervention can be instituted.

Sheldon[28] reported the following predisposing factors for a poor bereavement outcome:

- Ambivalent or dependent relationship
- Multiple prior bereavements
- Previous mental illness, especially depression, and low self-esteem

Predisposing factors at time of death include:

- A sudden and unexpected death
- Death of a young person
- Lack of preparation for the death
- Stigmatized deaths (e.g., AIDS, suicide, culpable death)
- Sex of the bereaved person (e.g., elderly male widower), caring for the deceased person for >6 months
- Inability to carry out valued religious rituals

Boyle, Feng, and Raab[29] reaffirm that widowhood increases the risk of death regardless of the type of death of the spouse, noting that the risk of mortality is increased 10%–40% for the surviving spouse.

After the death, such factors as level of perceived social support, hardiness, lack of opportunities for new interests, and stress from other life crises—as well as dysfunctional behaviors and attitudes appearing early in the bereavement period, consumption of alcohol and drugs, smoking, morbid guilt, and the professional caregiver's gut feeling that this patient will not do well—are predictive of poor outcomes.[28,29] Knowledge of and alertness to such predisposing factors are useful for the provision of help, both lay and professional, early in the course of the bereavement so as to prevent further debilitating events. In addition to social support, health-care policy can have a profound effect on the experience of bereavement as part of the context in which care is provided.[30]

Grief

Grief is a process. Grief begins before the death for the patient and survivor as they anticipate and experience the loss. Grief continues for the survivor with the loss of their loved one. The grief process is not always orderly and predictable. Freud's view that grief is a normal process and that "a lost love object is never totally relinquished" is congruent with current thinking.[31] The initiation of the modern study of death and dying, however, especially in America, is often attributed to Erich Lindemann, a physician at the Massachusetts General Hospital, who responded to the survivors of a fire in Boston's Coconut Grove nightclub. Five hundred persons died as a result of the fire, which took place on Thanksgiving eve, 1942. Lindemann, a psychiatrist, was interested at the time in the emotional reaction of patients to body disfigurement and plastic surgery.[32] With this medical interest, "Lindemann was struck by the similarity of responses between his patients' reactions to facial disfigurement or loss of a body part and the reactions of the survivors of the fire."[32(p105)]

This observation led Lindemann to a study of 101 patients including psychoneurotic patients who lost a relative during the course of treatment; relatives of patients who died in the hospital; bereaved disaster victims (Coconut Grove fire) and their close relatives; and relatives of members of the armed forces.[33] Based on the study of these patients, he determined **five indicators that are "pathognomonic for grief"**[33]:

1. Sensations of somatic distress, such as tightness in the throat, choking, and shortness of breath
2. Intense preoccupation with the image of the deceased
3. Strong feelings of guilt
4. A loss of warmth toward others with a tendency to respond with irritability and anger
5. Disoriented behavior patterns

Lindemann used the term "grief work" to describe the process by which individuals attempt to adjust to their loss.[33]

Various theorists have developed a series of stages and phases of grief work. Kübler-Ross[34] identified five stages:

1. Denial and isolation
2. Anger
3. Bargaining
4. Depression
5. Acceptance

The commonality among theorists of the stages of grief is that the individual moves through

1. Notification and shock,
2. Experience of the loss emotionally and cognitively, and
3. Reintegration.

Based on these stages or phases of grief, Corr and Doka[35] proposed the following grief work that needed to be done by the individual:

1. Share acknowledgment of the reality of death.
2. Share in the process of working through the pain of grief.
3. Reorganize the family system.
4. Restructure the family's relationship with the deceased and reinvest in other relationships and life pursuits.

Areas of Disagreement Around Grief Work

1. *The degree to which separation from the deceased must occur.* Klass and associates[36] argue that such bonds continue. They suggest that "survivors hold the deceased in loving memory for long periods, often forever," and that maintaining an inner representation of the deceased is normal. Winston's study of African American grandmothers demonstrated that they maintained strong bonds with the deceased.[37]

2. *An expectation that intense grief must be resolved within a given time frame,* such as 2 weeks, and whether the concept of recovery, or some other term, best connotes what occurs after coming to terms with a death and getting on with one's life.[38,39]

3. *The concept of recovery.* It has been suggested that "recovery" is a term more appropriate to an illness, and that death is a normal process of life. Balk[40] argues for a term that incorporates the potential for transformative growth.

4. *Medicalization of the grief process.* Given that death is a normal part of the cycle of living, grief too is considered a normal process. However, grief although a normal part of life, may also become "complicated." As such, interventions may be needed.

5. *Efficacy of grief counseling.* Larson and Hoyt[41] argue that the pessimistic view of the value of grief counseling is unfounded.

Types of Grief

The types of grief discussed below are not exhaustive of all types of grief, but rather encompass the major categories. Different terms such as "common grief" and "chronic grief" may be used for some of the same phenomena.

Anticipatory Grief

Anticipatory grief is the grief experienced before the actual loss. It is associated with diagnosis, acute and chronic illness, and terminal illness experienced by the patient, family, and caregivers. Examples of anticipatory grief include actual or potential fear of loss of health; loss of independence; loss of a body part; loss of financial stability, loss of choice, or loss of mental function. Byrne and Raphael[42] found that "widowers who were unable to anticipate their wife's death, even when their wife had suffered a long final illness, had a more severe bereavement reaction." Anticipatory grief is unconscious preparation for status change and is not a conscious, deliberative process. The term "premature grief" has also been given to this process.[43]

Anticipatory grief is distinguished from the concept of **forewarning**. An example of forewarning is learning of a terminal diagnosis. Anticipatory grief is an unconscious process, whereas forewarning is a conscious process. Even with forewarning, preparation for loss may not occur, as it may be perceived as a betrayal of the terminally ill person.

If forewarning it is used to make some preparation for role change, such as becoming familiar with the intricacies of the role the terminally ill person plays in the family (e.g., mastering a checking account or other financial responsibilities of the family), such time may be used to the benefit of all concerned. In contrast, anticipatory grief resulting in reinvestment of emotional energy before the death of the terminally ill person is detrimental to the relationship.

Duke[44] interviewed five spouses in the second year of their bereavement. The research identified four areas of change: role change from spouse to caregiver during the illness, followed by loss of those roles in bereavement and needing to be cared for; relationship changes from being with spouse to being alone; coping changes from being in suspense to being in turmoil; and the change from experiencing and gathering memories to remembering and constructing memories.[44] These findings reflect the general changes that occur over a terminal illness and *not* the experience of anticipatory grief.

Uncomplicated Grief

Normal grief reactions to a loss can be physical, emotional, cognitive, and behavioral. Active grieving can take years. We do not get over the loss, but the relationship with the deceased changes. There is a reconnection with the world of the living. Worthington[45] depicted a linear model of uncomplicated grief based on adjustment. In this model, an individual in a normal emotional state experiences a loss that causes a reaction and an emotional low; subsequently, the individual begins a recovery to his or her former state. This process of recovery is occasioned by brief periods of relapse, but not to the depths experienced previously. Ultimately, the individual moves to adjustment to the loss.

Niemeyer[46] offered a different perspective on grief, focusing on meaning reconstruction. He developed a set of propositions to capture adaptation to loss:

1. Death as an event can validate or invalidate the constructions that form the basis on which we live, or it may stand as a novel experience for which we have no constructions.

2. Grief is a personal process, one that is idiosyncratic, intimate, and inextricable from our sense of who we are.

3. Grieving is something we do, not something that is done to us.

4. Grieving is the act of affirming or reconstructing a personal world of meaning that has been challenged by loss.
5. Feelings have functions and should be understood as signals of the state of our meaning-making efforts.
6. We construct and reconstruct our identities as survivors of loss in negotiations with others.

Niemeyer[46] viewed meaning reconstruction as the central process of grief. The inability to make meaning could lead to complications.

Complicated Grief

There are four types of complicated grief:

Chronic grief is characterized by normal grief reactions that do not subside and continue over very long periods of time.

Delayed grief is characterized by normal grief reactions that are suppressed or postponed and the survivor consciously or unconsciously avoids the pain of the loss.

Exaggerated grief is where the survivor resorts to self-destructive behaviors.

Masked grief is where the survivor is not aware that behaviors that interfere with normal functioning are a result of the loss.

Risk factors for complicated grief include sudden or traumatic death, suicide, homicide, dependent relationship with the deceased, chronic illness, death of a child, multiple losses, unresolved grief from prior losses, concurrent stressors, difficult dying process such as pain and suffering, lack of support systems, and lack of a faith system.

In her discussion of complicated mourning, Rando[31] made observations applicable to complicated grief. She observed that, after a suitable length of time, the mourner is attempting to "deny, repress, or avoid aspects of the loss, its pain, and its implications and . . . to hold onto, and avoid relinquishing, the lost loved one. These attempts, or some variants thereof, cause the complications in mourning." These complications have also been noted to occur before death in the caregivers of cancer patients.[47]

Diagnostic criteria for complicated grief disorder include "the current experience (>1 year after a loss) of intensive intrusive thoughts, pangs of severe emotion, distressing yearnings, feeling excessively alone and empty, excessively avoiding tasks reminiscent of the deceased, unusual sleep disturbances, and maladaptive levels of loss of interest in personal activities." Some researchers have underscored the need to specify complicated grief as a unique disorder, and have developed an inventory of complicated grief to measure maladaptive symptoms of loss.[48] The Inventory of Complicated Grief is composed of 19 items with responses ranging from "Never" to "Rarely," "Sometimes," "Often," and "Always." Examples of items include, "I think about this person so much that it's hard for me to do the things I usually do"; "Ever since she (or he) died it is hard for me to trust people"; "I feel that it is unfair that I should live when this person died"; and "I feel lonely a great deal of the time ever since she (or he) died."[48] This inventory differentiates between complicated grief and depression.[48] Finally, it is the severity of symptomatology and the duration that distinguishes abnormal and complicated responses to bereavement.[49] Ruminative coping as an avoidance of grief work has been proposed as a variant of complicated chronic grief.[50]

The Inventory of Complicated Grief was used by Ott[51] with 112 bereaved participants in a study in which those identified as experiencing complicated grief were compared with those who were not. Those with complicated grief both identified more additional life stressors and felt they had less social support than the other bereaved individuals in the study. Lack of preparation for the death of a loved one has also been associated with complicated grief and depression.[52] The perspective of complicated grief as a stress response syndrome has been explicated by Shear and colleagues.[53] The characteristics of complicated grief have not been found to vary by race or by the violence of the loss.[54,55] Complicated grief may require professional intervention.[41,56] Approaches to therapy have included cognitive-behavioral therapy, presented face-to-face as well as over the Internet, and supportive counseling.[56–58]

Disenfranchised Grief

Doka[59] defined disenfranchised grief as "grief that results when a person experiences a significant loss and the resultant grief is not openly acknowledged, socially validated, or publicly mourned. In short, although the individual is experiencing a grief reaction, there is no social recognition that the person has a right to grieve or a claim on social sympathy or support." Those who are grieving the loss of relationships that may not be publicly acknowledged are not accorded the deference and support usually afforded the bereaved. Nonsanctioned relationships, either heterosexual or homosexual, may result in the exclusion of individuals not legitimated by blood or legal union.[60] A 2007 study underscores the finding of less social support for the bereaved spouses of same-sex couples.[61] However, the norms of society change, and the US Supreme Court ruling in June 2015 legalized same-sex marriage nationwide. Same-sex couples were accorded the same recognition as opposite-sex couples at the federal and state/territory level. Although the law is clear, the ruling is controversial among some segments of society and it will take time before being fully integrated into society. The AIDS quilt has done much to provide a public mourning ritual, but had not alleviated the disenfranchised status of some homosexual or lesbian partners. The result is what has been termed "modulated mourning."[60] This response to stigmatization constrains the public display of mourning by the griever. In this situation, the griever is not recognized.[62] The griever with intellectual disabilities may also not be recognized.[63]

Other instances in which a loss has not been legitimized include ex-spouses or ex-partners; friends, lovers, mistresses, or coworkers; mother of a stillborn child; and women (and husbands/boyfriends, lovers) who have experienced a terminated pregnancy. Loss resulting from miscarriage or abortion has only recently been recognized. In Japan, a "cemetery" is devoted to letters written by families each year telling miscarried or aborted children about the important events that occurred in the family that year and also expressing continued grief at their loss. Grieving in secret is a burden that makes the process more difficult to complete. Disenfranchised grief may also be a harbinger of unresolved grief.

Unresolved Grief

Unresolved grief is a failure to accomplish the necessary grief work. A variety of factors may give rise to unresolved grief, including guilt, loss of an extension of the self, reawakening of an old loss, multiple losses, inadequate ego development, and idiosyncratic resistance to mourning.[64(pp64–65)] In addition to these psychological factors, such social factors as social negation of a loss, socially unspeakable loss, social isolation and/or geographic distance from social support, assumption of the role of the strong one, and uncertainty over the loss (e.g., a disappearance at sea) may be implicated in unresolved grief.[64(pp66–67)] By helping significant others express their feelings and complete their business before the death of a loved one, unresolved grief and the accompanying manifestations can be prevented to some extent.

Eakes and coworkers[65] questioned whether "closure" is a necessary outcome of grief work. They explored the concept of "chronic sorrow" in bereaved individuals who experienced episodic bouts of sadness related to specific incidents or significant dates. These authors suggested the fruitfulness of maintaining an open-ended model of grief. With this in mind, grief is always unresolved to some degree; this is not considered pathological but rather an acknowledgment of a death. This theory is the chronic sorrow model.[66]

Expressions of Grief

Expressions of grief within the range considered normal in this society are described in the following section. It is important to note that what is considered appropriate in one group may be considered deviant or even pathological in another.

Symptoms of Grief

The manifestations of grief and bereavement are influenced by culture.[67] Intense grieving beyond 2 weeks in duration is considered in need of psychiatric intervention.[68] Some professionals in the field consider such an approach as ill-advised and inappropriate "Death is a life-altering event, but grief is not a pathological condition."[69] Balk and colleagues state, "We are concerned that for reasons of economic profit and clinical efficiency, people will often be prematurely diagnosed with depression and put on medication, rather than offered person-to-person counseling."[70(p208)] Wakefield warns against pathologizing grief when he states that the "grief process is less a step-wise preset series of events that lead to full resolution of pain, as classically portrayed, and more an individually constructed compromise between a degree of pain that never fully resolves and the need to compartmentalize that pain to move on with one's life."[71(p509)] Wakefield concurs with Bowlby that "normal grief can be a very lengthy process."[71]

Table 2.1 Manifestations of Grief

Physical	Cognitive	Emotional	Behavioral
Headaches	Sense of depersonalization	Anger	Impaired work performance
Dizziness	Inability to concentrate	Guilt	Crying
Exhaustion	Sense of disbelief and confusion	Anxiety	Withdrawal
Muscular aches	Idealization of the deceased	Sense of helplessness	Avoiding reminders of the deceased
Sexual impotency	Search for meaning of life and death	Sadness	Seeking or carrying reminders of the deceased
Loss of appetite	Dreams of the deceased	Shock	
Insomnia	Preoccupation with image of deceased	Yearning	Overreactivity
Feelings of tightness or hollowness	Fleeting visual, tactile, olfactory, auditory hallucinatory experiences	Numbness	Changed relationships
Breathlessness		Self-blame	
Tremors		Relief	
Shakes			
Oversensitivity to noise			

Source: Adapted from Doka[72]

Physical, Cognitive, Emotional, and Behavioral Symptoms of Grief[72]

Table 2.1 is not exhaustive of all of potential symptoms, but rather is illustrative of the expressions and manifestations of grief. What distinguishes "normal" grief from complicated grief is that it is usually self-limited. Although manifestations of grief at 1, 3, and 15 months after the death are not the same in intensity, a recent paper on grieving widows found the widows, while experiencing a decline in symptomatology, also continued experiencing symptoms for up to 5 years.[73]

A bereavement assessment tool links five questions to be asked of the bereaved to Maslow's hierarchy of needs.[74] The five questions address physiological, safety, belongingness, esteem, and self-actualization needs. No clinical or research data is provided on the use of the hierarchy of needs in this way.

Mourning Rituals

O'Gorman contrasted death rituals in England with those in Ireland. She recalled the "Protestant hushed respectfulness which had somehow infiltrated and taken over a Catholic community."[75(p1133)] The body was taken from the home by the funeral director. Children continued with school and stayed with relatives; they were shielded from the death. By way of contrast, in an Irish wake, "The body, laid out by a member of the family in order to receive a 'special blessing,' would be in the parlor of a country house surrounded by flowers from the garden and lighted candles."[75(p1133)] The children, along with the adult members of the family, viewed the corpse. "When visitors had paid their last respects they would join the crowd in the kitchen, who would then spend all night recounting stories associated with the dead person."[75(p1133)] O'Gorman noted the plentiful availability of alcohol and stated, "by the end of the night, to the uninitiated the event would appear to be more like a party than a melancholy event."[75(p1133)] Although O'Gorman initially found this distasteful, she "now believes that rituals like the Irish wake celebrate death as a happy occasion and bestow grace upon those leaving life and upon a community of those who mourn them."[75(p1133)]

The Irish wake, like the reception held in a church basement, hall, restaurant, or private home, serves not only for the expression of condolences but also as an opportunity to reinforce the connections of the community. The good send-off is part of the function of the funeral as a particular rite—that is, as a means of atoning for the sins of the mortal being, and as preparation for life in the afterworld.[76] Fulton noted two other functions of funerals, namely integration and separation. The former concerns the living; the latter refers to separation from the loved one as a mortal person.[72,76]

In the United States, funeral services are held not only in religious establishments such as churches or synagogues, but also in funeral homes. These services, frequently under the aegis of a clergyperson, may also be conducted by a staff member of the funeral home. More recently these services have also taken on the earmarks of a memorial service, accompanied by pictures of the deceased and the bereaved and remarks by selected close family members and friends of the deceased. In Judaism, the assumption is that the bereaved are to focus on their loss and the grieving of that loss. They are to pay no attention to worldly considerations. This period of time of exemption from customary roles may facilitate the process. Certainly having a "minion," in which 10 men and women (10 men for Orthodox Jews) say prayers each evening, reinforces the reality of the death and the separation. For the Orthodox, the mourning period is 1 year.[77]

A very different pattern is practiced by the Hopi in Arizona. The Hopi have a brief ceremony with the purpose of completing the funeral as quickly as possible so as to get back to customary activities.[77] The fear of death and the dead, and of spirits, induces distancing by the Hopi from nonliving phenomena. Stroebe and Stroebe[77] contrasted Shinto and Buddhist mourners in Japan with the Hopi. Both Shinto and Buddhist mourners practice ancestor worship; as a result, the bereaved can keep contact with the deceased, who become ancestors. Speaking to ancestors as well as offering food is accepted practice. In contrast to this Japanese practice, what occurs in the United States is that those bereaved who speak with a deceased person do so quietly, hiding the fact from others, believing others will consider it suspect or pathological. It is, however, a common occurrence. As mentioned previously, bringing food to the ancestor, or (e.g., to celebrate the Day of the Dead) to the cemetery, is part of the mourning practice in Hispanic and many other societies.

Practices, however, change with time, although one can often find the imprint of earlier rituals. The practice of saving a lock of hair or the footprint of a deceased newborn may have evolved from the practice in Victorian times of using hair for mourning brooches and lockets.[78] Mitchell and colleagues suggest that "virtual memorials blur the boundaries between the living and the dead."[79(p426)] These mourning practices of virtual memorials provide continuing bonds with the deceased.

Bereavement Support

Formal support, as an addition to support from one's social network has been found to be useful by some. Diamond and colleagues[80] demonstrate the utility of such outside support particularly for those not wanting to burden family and friends.

Formal Support

Many of the mourning practices noted previously provide support by the community to the bereaved (Table 2.2).

Other examples of formal support include support groups such as the widow-to-widow program and the Compassionate Friends for families of deceased children. The widow-to-widow program provides a formal mechanism for sharing one's emotions and experience with individuals who have had a similar experience. The Widowed Persons Service offers support for men and women via self-help support groups and a variety of educational and social activities. The Compassionate Friends, also a self-help organization, seeks to help parents and siblings after the death of a child. Other support groups may or may not have the input of a professional to run the group.

Table 2.2 Bereavement Practices	
Lay	**Professional**
1. Friendly visiting	1. Clergy visiting
2. Provision of meals	2. Clergy counseling
3. Informal support by previously bereaved	3. Nurse, MD, psychologist, social worker, psychiatrist counseling
4. Lay support groups	4. Professionally led support groups
5. Participation in cultural and religious rituals	5. Organization of memorial services by hospice and palliative care organizations
6. A friendly listener	6. A thoughtful listener
7. Involvement in a cause-related group	7. Referral to individuals with similar cause-related concerns
8. Exercise	8. Referral to a health club
9. Joining a new group	9. Referral to a bereavement program

Formal programs for children's bereavement support include peer support programs and art therapy programs. Institutions with bereavement programs, whether for children or adults, often send cards at the time of a patient's death, on the birthday of the deceased, and at 3, 6, 12, and 24 months after the death. Pamphlets with information about grief, a bibliography of appropriate readings, and contact numbers of support groups are also helpful. Family bereavement programs have been found to lead to improved parenting, coping, and caregiver mental health. The provision of bereavement follow-up to parents who have experienced the loss of a child or a pregnancy loss is helpful to the parents and also has implications for the support of the nurses and others who deliver this service.[81]

Attention to staff bereavement support has been given by institutional trauma programs, in emergency departments, and in critical care departments.[82] Brosche[83] provides a description of a grief team within a healthcare system. Keene, Hutton, Hall, and Rushton[84] outline a format for bereavement debriefing. This attention to the grief of healthcare providers empowers those involved to express their grief rather than to suppress it. All of these programs, whether for healthcare providers or family and significant others, maintain contact with the bereaved so as to provide support and make referrals to pastoral care personnel and other professionals as needed.

A variety of approaches have been used in working with the bereaved. Indeed, the combination of "religious psychotherapy" and a cognitive-behavioral approach was observed to be helpful to highly religious bereaved persons.[85] Religious psychotherapy for a group of Malays who adhered to the religion of Islam consisted of discussion and reading of verses of the Koran and Hadith, the encouragement of prayers, and a total of 12 to 16 psychotherapy sessions.[85] A bereavement support group intervention was demonstrated to have a significant impact on the grief of homosexual men who were or were not seropositive for the human immunodeficiency virus (HIV-1).[86] The need for support was found to be all the more necessary for bereaved women living with HIV, who "may be at increased risk for bereavement complicated with psychiatric morbidity and thoughts of suicide."[87(p225)] The risk-reduction effects of a community bereavement support program for HIV-positive individuals was demonstrated by a community support program in Ontario, Canada.[88] These outcomes have implications for the approaches nurses use with other bereaved clients.

Support groups may be open ended (i.e., without a set number of sessions), or they may be closed and limited to a particular set of individuals. Support groups with a set number of sessions have a beginning and end and are therefore more likely to be closed to new members until a new set of sessions begins. Open-ended groups have members who stay for varying lengths of time and may or may not have a topic for each session. Lev and McCorkle[89] found short-term programs of two to seven sessions, or meeting as needed, were the most effective. Other formal support entails working with a therapist or other healthcare provider (bereavement counseling). For those who were bereaved as a result of a suicide, the 6- to 8-week programs run by the Lifeline Community Care Group Brisbane helped to normalize the suicide bereavement experience.[18] Cloyes and colleagues[90] caution that the style of the interaction whether directive or facilitative has an impact on the opportunity for expression by the family caregiver. Arnold[91] suggested that the nurse should follow a process to assess the meaning of loss, the nature of the relationship, expressions and manifestations of grief, previous experience with grief, support systems, ability to maintain attachments, and progression of grief. Arnold underscored the importance of viewing grief as a healing process (Box 2.1). She gave the following example of a patient situation and two different approaches to diagnosis[91]:

A newly widowed woman feels awkward about maintaining social relationships with a group of married couples with whom she had participated with her husband.

- Grief as a pathological diagnosis: social isolation *versus*
- Grief as a healthy diagnosis: redefinition of social support.[91]

In addition to conventional talking therapy, such techniques as letter writing, empty chair, guided imagery, and journal writing can be used (Table 2.3).

In letter writing, the empty chair technique, and guided imagery, the bereaved are encouraged to express feelings about the past or about what life is like without the deceased. These techniques can be helpful as the

Box 2.1 Assessment of Grief

The bereaved often are weary from caring for the deceased. During this period they may not have looked after themselves. An assessment should include:

1. A general health checkup and assessment of somatic symptoms
2. A dental visit
3. An eye checkup as appropriate
4. Nutritional evaluation
5. Sleep assessment
6. Examination of ability to maintain work and family roles
7. Determination of whether there are major changes in presentation of self
8. Assessment of changes resulting from the death and the difficulties with these changes
9. Assessment of social networks

The healthcare worker needs to bear in mind that there is no magic formula for grieving. The key question is whether the bereaved is able to function effectively. Cues to the need for assistance include:

1. Clinical depression
2. Prolonged deep grief
3. Extreme grief reaction
4. Self-destructive behavior
5. Increased use of alcohol and/or drugs
6. Preoccupation with the deceased to exclusion of others
7. Perceived lack of social supports

"wish I had said" becomes said. A journal is also a vehicle for recording ongoing feelings of the lived experience of bereavement.

Grief is not pathology. It is a normal process that is expressed in individual ways. The techniques in Table 2.3 may prove helpful to the individual who is experiencing guilt about things not said or done. Another part of bereavement counseling is the instillation or reemergence of hope. As Cutcliffe[92] concluded, "There are many theories of bereavement counseling, with commonalities between these theories. While the theories

Table 2.3 **Counseling Interventions**	
1. Letter writing	The bereaved writes a letter to the deceased expressing the thoughts and feelings that may or may not have been expressed.
2. Empty chair	The bereaved sits across from an empty chair on which the deceased is imagined to be sitting. The bereaved is encouraged to express his or her feelings.
3. Empty chair with picture	A picture of the deceased is placed on the chair to facilitate the expressions of feelings by the bereaved.
4. Therapist assumes role of the deceased	In this intervention, the therapist helps the bereaved to explore his or her feelings toward the deceased by participating in a role-play.
5. Guided imagery	This intervention demands a higher level of skill than, for example, letter writing. Guided imagery can be used to explore situations that require verbalization by the bereaved to achieve completion. Imagery can also be used to recreate situations of dissension with the goal of achieving greater understanding for the bereaved.
6. Journal writing	This technique provides an ongoing vehicle for exploring past situations and current feelings. It is a helpful intervention to many.
7. Drawing pictures	For the artistically and not so artistically inclined, drawing pictures and explaining their content is another vehicle for discussing feelings and concerns.
8. Analysis of role changes	Helping the bereaved obtain help with the changes secondary to the death, such as with balancing a checkbook or securing reliable help with various home needs; assists with some of the secondary losses with the death of a loved one.
9. Listening	The bereaved has the need to tell his or her story. Respectful listening and concern for the bereaved is a powerful intervention that is much appreciated.
10. Venting anger	The professional can suggest the following:
	• Banging a pillow on the mattress. If combined with screaming, it is the best to do with the windows closed and no one in the home.
	• Screaming—at home or parked in a car in an isolated spot with the windows closed.
	• Crying—at home, followed by a warm bath and cup of tea or warm milk.
11. Normality barometer	Assuring the bereaved that the distress experienced is normal is very helpful to the bereaved.

indicate implicitly the re-emergence of hope in the bereft individual as a result of the counseling, they do not make specific reference to how this inspiration occurs." Cutcliffe saw the clear need to understand this process. In her exposition of the concept "hope," Stephenson[93] noted the association made by Frankl[94] between hope and meaning. Stephenson stated, "Frankl equated hope with having found meaning in life, and lack of hope as [having] no meaning in life."[93] Meaning-making appears key to the emergence of hope, and hope has been associated with coping.

In hospice programs, healthcare providers encourage dying persons and their families to have hope for each day. This compression of one's vision to the here and now may also be useful for the person who is grieving the loss of a loved one. Hope for the future and a personal future is the process that Cutcliffe[92] wished to elucidate. It may be a process that is predicated on hope for each day and having found meaning for the past.

A therapist provides a vehicle for ongoing discussion of the loss that informal caregivers may be unable to provide. A support group of bereaved individuals, or periodic contact by an institutional bereavement service, may also prove useful. What is helpful depends on the individual and his or her needs and also on the informal support that is available.

Informal Support

Informal support that is perceived as supportive and helpful can assist the bereaved to come to terms with life after the death of the beloved. Strategies evaluated as being helpful include "presence ('being there'), expressing the willingness to listen, and expressing care and concern, whereas the least positively evaluated strategies included giving advice, and minimization of other's feelings."[95(p419)] Whether the bereaved is isolated, or is part of a family or social group, is of tremendous import to the physical, psychological, and social welfare of the individual. Community in a psychosocial sense and a continuing role in the group are key factors in adjustment.

In societies where the widow has no role without her husband, she is figuratively if not literally disposed of in one way or another. It is for this reason that the woman who is the first in her group to experience widowhood has a much more difficult social experience than a woman who is in a social group where several women have become widows. In the former there is no reference group; in the latter there is.

The presence of family and friends takes on added significance after the initial weeks following the funeral. In those initial weeks, friendly visiting occurs with provision of a variety of types of foods considered appropriate in the group. After the initial period, friendly visiting is likely to decrease, and bereaved individuals may find themselves alone or the objects of financial predators. The counsel by the healthcare provider, or by family and friends, not to make life-altering decisions (e.g., moving) at this time unless absolutely necessary continues to be valuable advice. On the other hand, the comment that "time makes it easier" is a half-truth that is not perceived as helpful by the bereaved.[96]

Examples of what is helpful to the bereaved are—listening to music enjoyed by both the deceased and the bereaved[97] and being listened to by an interested person. Having family members with whom to grieve has been shown to be significant to the process of grief processing, and may enhance family bonding.[96] Quinton disliked the term "counseling" in that it implies the availability of a person with good counsel to confer. What Quinton considered important was "lots of listening to what the victim wants to off-load."[98(p32)] She observed, "The turning point for me was realizing that I had a right to feel sad, and to grieve and to feel miserable for as long as I felt the need."[98(p32)] By owning the grieving process, Quinton provided herself with the most important support for her recovery from a devastating experience—her mother's murder in a massacre by the Irish Republican Army in 1987. The lesson is applicable, however, to any bereaved person regardless of whether the death was traumatic or anticipated.

Is Grief Work Ever Completed?

As long as life and memory persist, the deceased individual remains part of the consciousness of family and friends. Lindemann's concept of grief work,[32,33] indicates that sooner or later that work needs to be accomplished. Delay protracts the time when accommodation is made. Grief work, however, is never over, in the sense that there will be moments in years to come when an occasion or an object revives feelings of loss. The difference is that the pain is not the same acute pain as that experienced when the loss initially occurred. How one arrives at the point of accommodation is a process termed "letting go."

Letting Go

The term "letting go" refers to acknowledgment of the loss of future togetherness—physical, psychological, and social. There is no longer a "we," only an "I" or a "we" without the deceased. Family members speak of events such as the first time a flower or bush blooms, major holidays, birthdays, anniversaries, and special shared times. Corless[99] quoted Jacqueline Kennedy, who spoke about "last year" (meaning 1962–1963) as the last time that her husband, John Kennedy, experienced a specific occasion:

> On so many days—his birthday, an anniversary, watching his children running to the sea—I have thought, "but this day last year was his last to see that." He was so full of love and life on all those days. He seems so vulnerable now, when you think that each one was a last time.

Mrs. Kennedy also wrote about the process of accommodation, although she didn't call it that[60]:

> Soon the final day will come around again—as inexorably as it did last year. But expected this time. It will find some of us different people than we were a year ago. Learning to accept what was unthinkable when he was alive changes you.

Finally, she addressed an essential truth of bereavement:

> I don't think there is any consolation. What was lost cannot be replaced.[99]

Letting go encompasses recognizing the uniqueness of the individual. It also entails finding meaning in the relationship and experience. It does not require cutting oneself off from memories of the deceased. It does require accommodating to the loss and to the continuing bonds with the deceased.

Continuing Bonds

Klass and associates[36] contributed to reformulation of thinking on the nature of accommodating to loss. Although it was postulated that the grief process should be completed in 1 year, when emotional energies would once again be invested in the living, the experience of the bereaved suggested otherwise. They maintain the presence of the deceased in their lives in a variety of different ways—some shared and some solitary.

Summary

A Turkish expression in the presence of death is, "May you live."[100] That indeed is the challenge of bereavement.

References

1. Lee RA, Whiting JB. Foster children's expressions of ambiguous loss. Am J Fam Ther. 2007;35:117–128. doi: 10, 1080/ 0192618060/057499.

2. Kagawa-Singer M. The cultural context of death rituals and mourning practices. Oncol Nurs Forum. 1998;25:1752.

3. Durkheim E. The Elementary Forms of Religious Life. New York: Collier; 1961.

4. DeSpelder LA, Strickland AL. The Last Dance. 9th ed. Mountain View, CA: Mayfield; 2011:207.

5. Kotze E. "Women . . . mourn and men carry on": African women storying mourning practices: a South African example. Death Stud. 2012;36:742–766.

6. Lee R, Vaughn M. Death and dying in the history of South Africa since 1800. JAH. 2008;49:341–359.

7. Bachelor P. Practical bereavement. Health Soc Rev. 2007;16: 405–414.

8. Yalom V. 2010. Kenneth Doka on Grief Counseling and Psychotherapy. http://www.psychotherapy.net/interview/grief-counseling-doka.

9. Rodgers L. Meaning of bereavement among older African-American widows. Geriatr Nurs. 2004;25:10–16.

10. Stroebe M, Schut H, Stroebe W. Health outcomes of bereavement. Lancet. 2007;370:1960–1973.

11. Zisook S, Kendler KS. Is bereavement-related depression different than non-bereavement-related depression? Psychol Med. 2007;37:779–794.

12. Middleton W, Franzp MD, Raphael B, Franzp MD, Burnett P, Martinek N. Psychological distress and bereavement. J Nerv Ment Dis. 1997;447–453.

13. Hays JC, Kasl S, Jacobs S. Past personal history of dysphoria, social support, and psychological distress following conjugal bereavement. J Am Geriatr Soc. 1994;42:712–718.

14. Zisook S, Shuchter SR, Sledge PA, Paulus M, Judd LL. The spectrum of depressive phenomena after spousal bereavement. J Clin Psychiatry. 1994;55(Suppl):29–35.

15 Rubin SS, Malkinson R, Witztum E. Working with the Bereaved: Multiple Lenses on Loss and Mourning. New York: Routledge Taylor & Francis; 2012.

16. Schulz R, Herbert R, Boerner K. Bereavement after caregiving. Geriatrics. 2008;63:20–22.

17. Boelen PA, van den Bout J, de Keijser J. Traumatic grief as a disorder distinct from bereavement-related depression and anxiety: a replication study with bereaved mental health care patients. Am J Psychiatry. 2003;160:1339–1341.

18. Groos AD, Shakespeare-Finch J. Positive experiences for participants in suicide bereavement groups: a grounded theory model. Death Stud. 2013;37:1–24.

19. Todd S. Silenced grief: living with the death of a child with intellectual disabilities. J Intellect Disabil Res. 2007;51:637–648.

20. Reilly DE, Hastings RP, Vaughan FL, Huws JC. Parental bereavement and the loss of a child with intellectual disabilities: a review of the literature. Intellect Dev Disabil. 2008;46:27–43.

21. Beck E, Jones SJ. Children of the condemned: grieving the loss of a father to death row. Omega. 2008;56:191–215.

22. Hogan NS, DeSantis L. Things that help and hinder adolescent sibling bereavement. West J Nurs Res. 1994;16:137.

23. Grenklo TB, Kreicbergs U, Hauksdottir A, et al. Self-injury in teenagers who lost a parent to cancer: a nationwide, population-based, long-term follow-up. JAMA Pediatr. 2013;167:133–140. doi:10.1001/jamapediatrics.2013.430.

24. Fitzpatrick, TR. Bereavement among faculty members in a university setting. Soc Work Health Care. 2007;45:83–109.

25. Baddeley JL, Singer JA. Telling losses: personality correlates and functions of bereavement narratives. J Res Pers. 2008;42:421–438.

26. Anderson KL, Dimond MF. The experience of bereavement in older adults. J Adv Nurs. 1995;22:308–315.

27. Pector EA. Sharing losses online: do Internet groups benefit the bereaved? Int J Childbirth Educ. 2012;27:19–25.

28. Sheldon F. ABC of palliative care: bereavement. BMJ. 1998;316:456.

29. Boyle PJ, Feng Z, Raab GM. Does widowhood increase mortality risk?: Testing for selection effects by comparing causes of spousal death. Epidemiology. 2011;22:1–5. doi:10.1097/EDE.06013e3181fdcc0b.

30. Holtslander LF. Caring for bereaved family caregivers: analyzing the context of care. Clin J Onc Nurs. 2008;510–506.

31. Rando TA. Grief and mourning: accommodating to loss. In: Wass H, Neimeyer RA, eds., Dying: Facing the Facts. Philadelphia: Taylor and Francis; 1995:211–241.

32. Fulton R, Bendikson R. Introduction: grief and the process of mourning. In: Fulton R, Bendicksen R, eds., Death and Identity. 3rd ed. Philadelphia: Charles Press; 1994:105–109.

33. Lindemann E. Symptomatology and management of acute grief. Am J Psychiatry. (Sesquicentennial Suppl) 1994;151(6):156.

34. Kübler-Ross E. On Death and Dying. New York: Macmillan, 1969.

35. Corr CA, Doka KJ. Current models of death, dying and bereavement. Crit Care Nurs Clin North Am. 1994;6:545–552.

36. Klass D, Silverman P, Nickman S. Continuing Bonds. Philadelphia: Taylor and Francis; 1996.

37. Winston CA. African American grandmothers parenting AIDS orphans: concomitant grief and loss. Am J Orthopsychiatry. 2003;73:91–100.

38. Shapiro ER. Whose recovery of what?: Relationships and environments promoting grief and growth. Death Stud. 2008;32(1):40–58.

39. Rosenblatt PC. Recovery following bereavement: metaphor, phenomenology, and Culture. Death Stud. 2008;32(1):6–16.

40. Balk DE. A modest proposal about bereavement and recovery. Death Stud. 2008;32(1):84–93.

41. Larson DG, Hoyt WT. What has become of grief counseling?: An evaluation of the empirical foundations of the new pessimism. Prof Psychol Res Pract. 2007;38:347–355.

42. Byrne GJA, Raphael B. A longitudinal study of bereavement phenomena in recently widowed elderly men. Psychol Med. 1994;23:411–421.

43. Grassi L. Bereavement in families with relatives dying of cancer. Curr Opin Support Palliat Care. 2007;1(1):43–49.

44. Duke S. An exploration of anticipatory grief: the lived experience of people during their spouses' terminal illness and in bereavement. J Adv Nurs. 1998;28:829–839.

45. Worthington RC. Models of linear and cyclical grief: different approaches to different experiences. Clin Pediatr. 1994;33:297–300.

46. Neimeyer RA. Meaning reconstruction and the experience of chronic loss. In: Doka KJ, Davidson J, eds., Living with Grief: When Illness Is Prolonged. Philadelphia: Taylor and Francis; 1997:159–176.

47. Tomarken A, Holland J, Schachter S, et al. Factors of complicated grief pre-death in caregivers of cancer patients. Psycho-Oncol. 2008;17:105–111.

48. Prigerson HG, Maciejewski PK, Reynolds CF III, et al. Inventory of complicated grief: a scale to measure maladaptive symptoms of loss. Psychiatry Res. 1995;59:65–79.

49. Boelen PA, van den Bout J. Complicated grief and uncomplicated grief are distinguishable constructs. Psychiatry Res. 2008;157:311–314.

50. Stroebe M, Boelen PA, van den Hout M, Stroebe W, Salemink E, van den Bout J. Ruminative coping as avoidance: a reinterpretation of its function in adjustment to bereavement. Eur Arch Psychiatry Clin Neurosci. 2007;257:462–472.

51. Ott CH. The impact of complicated grief on mental and physical health at various points in the bereavement process. Death Stud. 2003;27:249–272.

52. Loke AY, Li Q, Man LS. Preparing family members for the death of their loved one with cancer. J Hosp Palliat Nurs. 2013;15:E1–E11.

53. Shear K, Monk T, Houck P, et al. An attachment-based model of complicated grief including the role of avoidance. Eur Arch Psychiatry Clin Neurosci. 2007;257:453–461.

54. Cruz M, Scott J, Houck P, Reynolds CF, Frank E, Shear MK. Clinical presentation and treatment outcome of African Americans with complicated grief. Psychiatr Serv. 2007;58:700–702.

55. Boelen PA, van den Bout J. Examination of proposed criteria for complicated grief in people confronted with violent or nonviolent loss. Death Stud. 2007;31:155–164.

56. Shear MK, Simon N, Wall M, et al. Complicated grief and related bereavement issues for DSM-5. Depress Anxiety. 2011;28:103–117.

57. Boelen PA, de Keijser J, van den Hout M, van den Bout J. Treatment of complicated grief: a comparison between cognitive-behavioral therapy and supportive counseling. J Counsel Clin Psychol. 2007;75:277–284.

58 Wagner B, Maercker A. A 1.5-year follow-up of an Internet based intervention for complicated grief. J Trauma Stress. 2007;20:625–629.

59. Doka K. Disenfranchised grief in historical and cultural perspective. In: Stroebe M, Hansson RO, Schenk H, Stroebe W, van den Blink E, eds., Handbook of Bereavement Research and Practice: Advances in Theory and Intervention. Washington, DC: American Psychological Association; 2008:223–240.

60. Corless IB. Modulated mourning: The grief and mourning of those infected and affected by HIV/AIDS. In: Doka KJ, Davidson J, eds., Living with Grief: When Illness Is Prolonged. Philadelphia: Taylor and Francis; 1997:108–118.

61. Boswell C. A phenomenological study of the experience of grief resulting from spousal bereavement in heterosexual and homosexual men and women. A dissertation presented to the Faculty of the College of Education. University of Houston. 2007.

62. Gataric G, Kinsel B, Currie BG, Lawhorne LW. Reflections on the under-researched topic of grief in persons with dementia: a report from a symposium on grief and dementia. Am J Hosp Palliat Care. 2010;27:567–574. doi:10.1177/1049909110371315.

63. McEvoy J, MacHale R, Tierney E. Concept of death and perceptions of bereavement in adults with intellectual disabilities. J Intellect Disabil Res. 2012; 56;191–203.

64. Rando TA. Grief, Dying and Death: Clinical Interventions for Caregivers. Champaign, IL: Research Press, 1984.

65. Eakes GG, Burke ML, Hainsworth MA. Chronic sorrow: the experiences of bereaved individuals. Illness Crisis Loss. 1999;7:172–182.

66. Eakes GG, Burke ML, Hainsworth MA. Theory of chronic sorrow. In: Masters K, ed., Nursing Theories: A Framework for Professional Practice. Sudbury, MA: Jones and Bartlett Learning, 2010:349–361.

67. HardyBougere M. Cultural manifestations of grief and bereavement: a clinical perspective. J Cult Divers. 2008;15:66–69.

68. American Psychiatric Association. Diagnostic and Statistical Manual of Mental Disorders. 5th ed. Arlington, VA: American Psychiatric Publishing; 2013.

69. Attig T, Corless IB, Gilbert, KR, et al. When does a broken heart become a mental disorder? The Dougy Center: The National Center for Grieving Children and Families. http://www.dougy.org.

70. Balk DE, Noppe I, Sandler I, Werth J. Bereavement and depression: possible changes to the diagnostic and statistical manual of mental disorders: a report from the scientific advisory committee of the Association for Death Education and Counseling. Omega. 2011:63:199–220.

71. Wakefield JC. Should prolonged grief be reclassified as a mental disorder in DSM-5?: Reconsidering the empirical and conceptual arguments for complicated grief disorder. J Nerv Ment Dis. 2012:200:499–511. doi:10.1097/nmd.06013e3182482155.

72. Doka K. Grief. In: Kastenbaum R, Kastenbaum B, eds., Encyclopedia of Death. Phoenix, AZ: Oryx Press; 1989:127.

73. Kowalski SD, Bondmass MD. Physiological and psychological symptoms of grief in widows. Res Nurs Health. 2008;31:23–30.

74. Love AW. Progress in understanding grief, complicated grief, and caring for the bereaved. Contemp Nurse. 2007;27:73–83.

75. O'Gorman SM. Death and dying in contemporary society: an evaluation of current attitudes and the rituals associated with death and dying and their relevance to recent understandings of health and healing. J Adv Nurs. 1998;2:1127–1135.

76. Fulton R. The funeral in contemporary society. In Fulton R, Bendiksen R, eds., Death and Identity. 3rd ed. Philadelphia: Charles Press; 1994:288–312.

77. Stroebe W, Stroebe MS. Is grief universal?: Cultural variations in the emotional reaction to loss. In Fulton R, Bendiksen R, eds., Death and Identity. 3rd ed. Philadelphia: Charles Press; 1994:177–207.

78. Byatt AS. Possession: A Romance. New York: Vintage Books, 1990:6.

79. Mitchell LM, Stephenson PH, Cadell S, Macdonald, ME. Death and grief on-line: virtual memorialization and changing concepts of childhood death and parental bereavement on the Internet. Health Soc Rev. 2012; 21(4):413–431.

80. Diamond H, Llewelyn S, Relf M, Bruce C. Helpful aspects of bereavement support for adults following an expected death: volunteers' and bereaved people's perspectives. Death Stud. 2012;36:541–564.

81. MacConnell G, Aston M, Randel P, Zwaagstra N. Nurses' experiences providing bereavement follow-up: an exploratory study using feminist poststructuralism. J Clin Nurs. 2012;22:1094–1102. doi: 10.1111/j.1365-2702.2012.04272.x.

82. LeBrocq P, Charles A, Chan T, Buchanan M. Establishing a bereavement program: caring for bereaved families and staff in the emergency department. Accid Emerg Nurs. 2003;11:85–90.

83. Brosche TA. A grief team within a healthcare system. Dimens Crit Care Nurs. 2007;26:21–28.

84. Keene EA, Hutton N, Hall B, Rushton C. Bereavement debriefing sessions: an intervention to support health care professionals in managing their grief after the death of a patient. Pediatr Nurs. 2010; 36:185–189.

85. Azhar MZ, Varma SL. Religious psychotherapy as management of bereavement. Acta Psychiatr Scand. 1995;91:233–235.

86. Goodkin K, Blaney NT, Feaster DJ, Baldewicz T, Burkhalter JE, Leeds B. A randomized controlled clinical trial of a bereavement support group intervention in human immunodeficiency virus type 1-seropositive and -seronegative homosexual men. Arch Gen Psychiatry. 1999;56:52–59.

87. Sikkema KJ, Hansen NB, Kochman A, Tate DC, Difranceisco W. Outcomes from a randomized controlled trial of a group intervention for HIV positive men and women coping with AIDS-related loss and bereavement. Death Stud. 2004;28:187–209.

88. Leaver CA, Perreault Y, Demetrakopoulos A; AIDs Bereavement Project of Ontarios' Survive and Thrive Working Group. Understanding AIDS-related bereavement and multiple loss among long-term survivors of HIV in Ontario. Can J Hum Sex. 2008:17:37–52.

89. Lev EL, McCorkle R. Loss, grief and bereavement in family members of cancer patients. Semin Oncol Nurs. 1998;4:145–151.

90. Cloyes KG, Berry PH, Reblin M, Clayton M, Ellington L. Exploring communication patterns among hospice nurses and family caregivers. J Hosp Palliat Nurs. 2012;14:426–437. doi:10.1097/NJH.06013e318251598b.

91. Arnold J. Rethinking: nursing implications for health promotion. Home Healthc Nurse. 1996;14:779–780.

92. Cutcliffe JR. Hope, counselling, and complicated bereavement reactions. J Adv Nurs. 1998;28:760.

93. Stephenson C. The concept of hope revisited for nursing. J Adv Nurs. 1991;16:1456–1461.

94. Frankl V. Man's Search for Meaning: An Introduction to Logotherapy. New York: Simon and Schuster, 1959.

95. Rack JJ, Burleson BR, Bodie GD, Holmstrom AJ, Servaty-Seib H. Bereaved adults' evaluations of grief management messages: effects of message person centeredness, recipient individual differences, and contextual factors. Death Stud. 2008;32:399–427.

96. Pressman DL, Bonanno GA. With whom do we grieve?: Social and cultural determinants of grief processing in the United States and China. J Soc Pers Relat. 2007;24:729–746.

97. O'Callaghan CC, McDermott F, Hudson P, Zalcberg JR. Sound continuous bonds with the deceased: the relevance of music including preloss music therapy, for eight bereaved caregivers. Death Studies. 2013:37(2):101–125. doi: 10.1080/07481187.2011.617488.

98. Quinton A. Permission to mourn. Nurs Times. 1994;90:31–32.

99. Corless IB. And when famous people die. In: Corless IB, Germino BA, Pittman MA (eds.), A Challenge for Living: Dying, Death, and Bereavement. Boston: Jones & Bartlett; 1995:398.

100. [Commentary by newscaster on Turkish earthquake.] ABC News, 1999.

Chapter 3

Supporting Families in Palliative Care

Rose Steele and Betty Davies

Key Points

- Palliative care is patient and family centered care.
- The illness affects both patient and family, and patient and family characteristics affect the illness.
- Geographic and cultural factors influence who is considered as family and what is expected from them in the setting of illness.
- Families who have a terminally ill member are in transition.

This chapter addresses family-centered care as central to the philosophy of palliative care. Illness is incorporated into every aspect of family life. Family and illness can be considered a biopsychosocial model—the fit between family strengths and vulnerabilities in relation to the psychosocial demands over time of the illness. Geographic and cultural factors influence who is included as "family." Expectations of roles, patterns of behavior, and rules of emotional expression vary considerably. As a basis for offering optimal support to families in palliative care, the main focus of the chapter is on findings of a research program that prospectively examined the experiences of such families. Particular attention is paid to the transition of "fading away."

Who Is the Family?

The family is a group of individuals inextricably linked in ways that are constantly interactive and mutually reinforcing.[1,2] Family can mean direct blood relatives, relationships through an emotional commitment, or the group or person with whom an individual feels most connected.[3] Moreover, family in its fullest sense embraces all generations—past, present, future; those living, those dead, and those yet to be born. Shadows of the past and dreams of the future also contribute to the understanding of families.

Although palliative care programs are based on the principle that the family is the unit of care, in practice the family is often viewed as a group of individuals who can either prove helpful or resist efforts to deliver care. The best outcomes can be achieved if appropriate interventions are directed at the family members both individually and as a group.[4,5] It is important to understand how all family members perceive their experience and how their relationships fit together. Research has focused on the family's perceptions of their needs[6–9]; experiences and challenges faced[6–12]; adaptation and coping skills required for home care[6,11,13–16]; the supportiveness of nursing behaviors[17] or physician behaviors[18]; and satisfaction with care.[19] Though past research focused primarily on families of patients with cancer, family research on other diagnostic populations, such as Parkinson's disease,[20] cardiac disease,[21] motor neuron disease,[22] dementia,[23] and neurodegenerative diseases,[7] as well as advanced age[24] is becoming available. Family members expect health professionals to meet their own needs for information, emotional support, and assistance with care.[18] Recent research suggests that the most effective way to support family caregivers may be to help them be successful in their caregiving role rather than to focus on personal needs.[12]

As a basis for offering optimal support to families in palliative care, this chapter focuses on describing the findings of a nursing research program that prospectively examined the experiences of such families.[25] Nurses in a regional cancer center constantly had to attend to the needs of not only patients but also patients' families, particularly as they moved back and forth between hospital and home. In searching the literature for guidelines about family-centered care, they found that many articles were about the needs of patients and family members, about levels of family members' satisfaction with care, and about family members' perceptions of nurses, but nothing really described the families' experiences as they coped with the terminal illness of a beloved family member. The research study[25] included patients with advanced cancer, their spouses, and at least one of their adult children (>18 years of age). Since the completion of the original research, families with AIDS, Alzheimer's disease, and cardiac disease have provided anecdotal validation of the findings from their experiences. In addition, families of children with progressive, life-threatening illness have provided similar validation. The findings from this research program form the basis for the description that follows. References to additional research studies are also included to supplement and emphasize the ongoing development of knowledge in the field of family-centered end-of-life care.

The Transition of Fading Away

A common view is that transitions are initiated by change, by the start of something new. However, most transitions actually begin with endings.[26] This is true for families living with serious illness. The transition described as "fading away" described by families facing terminal illness began with the ending of life as they knew it. They came to realize that the ill family member was no longer living with cancer but was now dying from cancer. Despite the fact that family members had been told about the seriousness of the prognosis, and had experienced the usual ups and downs associated with the illness trajectory, for many the "gut" realization that the patient's death was inevitable occurred suddenly: "It struck me hard—it hit me like a bolt. Dad is not going to get better!" The awareness was triggered when family members saw, with "new eyes," a change in the patient's body or physical capacity, such as the patient's weight loss, extreme weakness, lack of mobility, or diminished mental capacity. Realizing that the patient would not recover, family members began the transition of fading away. As one patient commented, "My body has shrunk so much—the other day, I tried on my favorite old blue dress and I could see then how much weight I have lost. I feel like a skeleton with skin! I am getting weaker. . . . I just can't eat much now, I don't want to. I can see that I am fading. . . . I am definitely fading away."

The transition of fading away is characterized by seven dimensions: redefining, burdening, struggling with paradox, contending with change, searching for meaning, living day by day, and preparing for death. The dimensions do not occur in linear fashion; rather, they are interrelated and inextricably linked to one another. Redefining, however, plays a central role. All family members experience these dimensions, although patients, spouses, and children experience each dimension somewhat differently.

Redefining

Redefining involves a shift from "what used to be" to "what is now." It demands adjustment in how individuals see themselves and each other. Patients maintained their usual patterns for as long as possible and then began to implement feasible alternatives once they realized that their capacities were seriously changing. Joe, a truck driver, altered his identity over time: "I just can't do what I used to. I finally had to accept the fact that the seizures made it unsafe for me to drive." Joe requested to help out at his company's distribution desk. When he could no longer concentrate on keeping the orders straight, Joe offered to assist with supervising the light loading. One day, Joe was acutely aware he didn't have the energy to even sit and watch the others: "I couldn't do it anymore," Joe sighed. "I had reached the end of my work life and the beginning of the end of my life." Another patient, Cora, lamented that she used to drive to her son's home to babysit her toddler-aged grandchildren; then her son dropped the children off at her house to conserve the energy it took for her to travel; and now, her son has made other child care arrangements. He brings the children for only short visits because of her extreme fatigue. Both Joe and Cora, like the other patients, accepted their limitations with much sadness and a sense of great loss. Their focus narrowed, and they began to pay attention to details of everyday life that they had previously ignored or overlooked. Joe commented, "When I first was at home, I wanted to keep in touch with the guys at the depot; I wanted to know what was going on. Now, I get a lot of good just watching the grandkids out there playing in the yard."

Patients were eager to reinforce that they were still the same on the inside, although they acknowledged the drastic changes in their physical appearance. They often became more spiritual in their orientation to life and nature. As Joe said, "I always liked being outside—was never much of an office-type person. But, now, it seems I like it even more. That part of me hasn't changed even though it's hard for some of the fellas (at work) to recognize me now." When patients were able to redefine themselves as Joe did, they made the best of their situation, differentiating what parts of them were still intact. Joe continued, "Yeah, I like just being outside, or watching the kids. And, you know, they still come to their Grandpa when their toy trucks break down—I can pretty much always fix 'em." Similarly, Cora commented: "At least, I can still make cookies for when my family comes, although I don't make them from scratch anymore." Patients shared their changing perceptions with family members and others, who then were able to offer understanding and support.

> "Nothing's wrong with me, really. . . . We are being accredited this year. There's a lot to do to get ready for that." Ralph insisted on going into the office each day to prepare the necessary reports. His increasing confusion and inability to concentrate made his reports inaccurate and inadequate, but Ralph refused to acknowledge his limitations or delegate the work. Instead, his colleagues had to work overtime to correct Ralph's work after he left the office. According to Ralph's wife, anger and frustration were commonplace among his colleagues, but they were reluctant to discuss the issue with Ralph. Instead, they avoided conversations with Ralph, and he complained to his wife about his colleagues' lack of interest in the project.

Patients who were unable to redefine themselves in this way attempted to maintain their regular patterns despite the obvious changes in their capacity to do so. They ended up frustrated, angry, and feeling worthless. These reactions distanced them from others, resulting in the patients feeling alone and, sometimes, abandoned. Ralph, for example, was an educational administrator. Despite his deteriorating health, he insisted that he was managing without difficulty.

Supporting Families

For the most part, spouses took the patient's physical changes in stride. They attributed the changes to the disease, not to the patient personally, and as a result, they were able to empathize with the patient. Patients' redefining focused on themselves, the changes in their physical status and intrapersonal aspects; spouses' redefining centered on their relationship with the patient. Spouses did their best to "continue on as normal," primarily for the sake of the patient. In doing so, they considered alternatives and reorganized their priorities.

Wittenberg and colleagues[4] described the "reciprocity of suffering" that family members experience, which results from the physical and emotional distress that is rooted in their anguish of dealing with the impending death of the loved one, and in their attempt to fill new roles as caregivers. The degree to which family members experienced this phenomenon varied according to patients' redefining. When patients were able to redefine themselves, spouses had an easier time. Such patients accepted spouses' offers of support; patients and spouses were able to talk about the changes that were occurring. Spouses felt satisfied in the care that they provided. But when patients were less able to redefine, then spouses' offers of support were rejected or unappreciated. For example, Ralph's wife worried about his work pattern and its impact on his colleagues. She encouraged him to cut back, but Ralph only ignored her pleas and implied that she did not understand how important this accreditation was to the future of his school. Even when Ralph was no longer able to go to the office, he continued to work from home, frequently phoning his colleagues to supervise their progress on the report. His wife lamented, "For an educated man, he doesn't know much. I guess it's too late to teach an old dog new tricks."

In such situations, spouses avoided talking about or doing anything that reminded the patient of the changes he or she was experiencing but not acknowledging. The relationship between the spouse and patient suffered. Rather than feeling satisfied with their care, spouses were frustrated and angry, although often they remained silent and simply "endured" the situation. The ill person contributed significantly to the caregiver's ability to cope. Indeed, the ill person was not simply a passive recipient of care but had an impact on the experience of the caregiving spouse. Similarly, in their study of factors that influence family caregiving, Stajduhar and colleagues[27] found that the ill person contributed significantly to the capacity of the spouse to continue to provide care despite their experience of overwhelming emotional and physical strain. Caregivers drew strength from the dying person when the ill person accepted the impending death, had an understanding of the caregivers' needs, and had attitudes, values, and beliefs that sustained their caregivers.

Adult children also redefined the ill family member; they redefined their ill parent from someone who was strong and competent to someone who was increasingly frail. Children felt vulnerable in ways they had not previously experienced. Most often, children perceived that the changes in their ill parent were the result of disease and not intentional: "It's not my father doing this consciously." Younger adult children were particularly sensitive to keeping the situation private, claiming they wanted to protect the dignity of the patient, but seemed to want to protect their own sense of propriety. For example, one young woman in her early twenties was "devastated" when her father's urinary bag dragged behind him as he left the living room where she and her friends were visiting. It was difficult for some young adults to accept such manifestations of their parent's illness. Adolescents in particular had a difficult time redefining the situation. They preferred to continue on as if nothing was wrong and to shield themselves against any information that would force them to see the situation realistically.

When the ill parent was able to redefine to a greater degree, then children were better able to appreciate that death is part of life. They recognized their own susceptibility and vowed to take better care of their own health; older children with families of their own committed to spending more quality time with their children. Joe talked, although indirectly, with his son about the situation: "I won't be here forever to fix the kids' toys." Together, Joe and his son reminisced about how Joe had always been available to his son and grandchildren as "Mr. Fix-it." Joe's son valued his dad's active participation in his life and promised to be the same kind of father to his own sons. In contrast, when the ill parent was unable to redefine, then children tended to ignore the present. They attempted to recreate the past to construct happy memories they never had. In doing so, they often neglected their own families. Ralph's daughter described her dad as a "workaholic." Feeling as if she had never had enough time with her dad, she began visiting her parents daily, with suggestions of places she could take him. He only became annoyed with her unfamiliar, constant presence: "It's okay she comes over every day, but enough is enough."

The extent to which spouses and adult children commented on the important contribution made by the dying family member underscores the importance of relationships among and between family members in facilitating their coping with the situation of terminal illness.

Burdening

Feeling burden for their family is common among patients.[28] If patients see themselves as purposeless, dependent, and immobile, they have a greater sense of burdening their loved ones. The more realistically patients redefined themselves as their capacities diminished, the more accurate they were in their perceptions of burdening. They acknowledged other family members' efforts, appreciated those efforts, and encouraged family members to rest and take time to care for themselves. Patients who were less able to redefine themselves did not see that they were burdening other family members in any way. They denied or minimized the strain on others. As Ralph said during the last week of his life, "I can't do much, but I am fine really. Not much has changed. It's a burden on my wife, but not much. It might be some extra work. . . . She was a nursing aide, so she is used to this kind of work."

Most spouses acknowledged the "extra load" of caring for their dying partner, but indicated that they did not regard the situation as a "burden." They agreed that it is "just something you do for the one you love." Spouses did not focus on their own difficulties; they managed to put aside their own distress so that it would not have a negative impact on their loved one. They sometimes shared stories of loneliness and helplessness, but also stories of deepening respect and love for their partner. Again, spouses of patients who were able to redefine were energized by the patient's acknowledgment of their efforts and were inspired to continue on. Spouses of patients who were not able to redefine felt unappreciated, exhausted, and confessed to "waiting for the patient to die."

The literature provides a comprehensive description of the multidimensional nature of burden experienced by family caregivers, but little attention has been given to burdening felt by patients or adult children specifically.

Caregiver burden, usually by spouses, has been described in terms of physical burden, which includes fatigue and physical exhaustion, sleeplessness, and deterioration of health.[4,10–16] Social burden encompasses limited time for self and social stress related to isolation.[10–14] Regardless of the type of burden, however, most caregivers, including the ones in the fading away studies, expressed much satisfaction with their caregiving.[4,14] Despite feeling burdened, most caregivers would repeat the experience: "Yes, it was difficult and exhausting, and there were days I didn't think I could manage one more minute. But, if I had to do it over again, I would. I have no regrets for what I am doing."

Children, too, experienced burdening, but the source stemmed from the extra responsibilities involved in helping to care for a dying parent, superimposed on their work responsibilities, career development, and their own families. As a result, adult children of all ages felt a mixture of satisfaction and exhaustion. Their sense of burdening was also influenced by the ill parent's redefining—if the ill parent acknowledged their efforts, they were more likely to feel satisfaction. However, children's sense of burdening was also influenced by the state of health of the well parent. If that parent was also ill or debilitated, the burden on children was compounded. If children were able to prioritize their responsibilities so that they could pay attention to their own needs as well as helping both their parents, they felt less burdened. Children seemed less likely than their well parents to perceive caregiving as something they themselves would do. They did not have the life experience of a long-term relationship that motivated the spouses to care for their partners.

Supporting Family Caregivers

Finding effective ways to support family caregivers is critical. An increase in the proportion of elderly people in the population means growing numbers of people with chronic, life-threatening, or serious illness require care. The responsibility for the care of such individuals is increasingly being placed on families. Respite care is often suggested as a strategy for relieving burden in family caregivers.[6,20] Although respite and other resources or services should be offered to families, each family must decide what will actually be helpful to them. For some families, inpatient respite services during the last year of life may help relieve their burden, while other caregivers may experience feelings of guilt and increased stress because of worrying about the quality of care provided.[29] Caregivers may be supported in their role simply by knowing there are resources and support available to them, even if they do not make use of these resources.[6]

Potential factors influencing the success of respite care include the dynamics within the family, in particular between the patient and family caregivers. Support from informal and professional caregivers was found not to be sufficient to balance the stresses of caregiving.[27] The missing element may be internal to the family. These findings encourage greater exploration into respite care and its meaning to caregivers. Family members may value cognitive breaks during which they can remain within the caregiving environment, but physical separation from the caregiving environment may be valuable only if it contributes in some meaningful way to the caregiving.

Struggling With Paradox

Struggling with paradox stems from the fact that the patient is both living and dying. For patients, the struggle focuses on wanting to believe they will survive and knowing that they will not. On "good days," patients felt optimistic about the outcome; on other days, they succumbed to the inevitability of their approaching demise. Often, patients did not want to "give up" but at the same time were "tired of fighting." They wanted to "continue on" for the sake of their families but also wanted "it to end soon" so their families could "get on with their lives." Patients coped by hoping for miracles, fighting for the sake of their families, and focusing on the good days. As Joe said, "I like to think about the times when things are pretty good. I enjoy those days. But, on the bad days, when I'm tired, or when the pain gets the best of me, then I just wonder if it wouldn't be best to just quit. But you never know—maybe I'll be the one in a million who makes it at the last minute." He then added wryly, "Hmmm, big chance of that."

Spouses struggled with a paradox of their own: they wanted to care for and spend time with the patient, and they also wanted a "normal" life. They coped by juggling their time as best they could, and usually put their own life on hold. Spouses who tended to their own needs usually were less exhausted and reported fewer health problems than spouses who neglected their own needs. For years, Joe and his wife had been square dancers. They had not been dancing together for many months when his wife resumed going to "dance night as a sub" or to prepare the evening's refreshments. "Sometimes, I feel guilty for going and leaving Joe at home, but I know I need a break. When I did miss dance night, I could see I was getting really bitchy—I need to get out for a breather so I don't suffocate Joe."

Children struggled with hanging on and letting go to a greater extent than their parents. They wanted to spend time with their ill parent and also to "get on with their own lives." Feeling the pressure of dual loyalties (to their parents and to their own young families), the demands of both compounded the struggle that children faced.

Contending With Change

Those facing terminal illness in a family member experience changes in every realm of daily life—relationships, roles, socialization, and work patterns. The focus of the changes differed among family members. Patients faced changes in their relationships with everyone they knew. They realized that the greatest change of their life was underway and that life as they knew it would soon be gone. They tended to break down tasks into manageable pieces, and increasingly they focused inward. The greatest change that spouses faced was in their relationship with the patient. They coped by attempting to keep everything as normal as possible. Children contended with changes that were more all-encompassing. They could not withdraw as their ill parent did, nor could they prioritize their lives to the degree that their well parent could. They easily became exhausted. As Joe's son explained, "It's a real challenge coming by this often —I try to come twice a week and then bring the kids on the weekends. But I just got a promotion at work this year, so that's extra work too. Seems like I don't see my wife much—but she's a real trooper. Her dad died last year so she knows what it's like."

Searching for Meaning

Searching for meaning has to do with seeking answers to help in understanding the situation.[30] Patients tended to journey inward, reflect on spiritual aspects, deepen their most important connections, and become closer to nature: "The spiritual thing has always been at the back of my mind, but it's developing more. . . . When you're sick like that, your attitude changes toward life. You come not to be afraid of death."

Spouses concentrated on their relationship with the patient. Some searched for meaning through personal growth, whereas others searched for meaning by simply tolerating the situation. Some focused on spiritual growth, and others adhered rigidly to their religion with little, if any, sense of inner growth or insight. Joe's wife commented, "Joe and I are closer than ever now. We don't like this business, but we have learned to love each other even more than when we were younger—sickness is a hard lesson that way." In contrast, Ralph's wife said with resignation, "He's so stubborn—always has been. I sometimes wonder why I stayed. But, here I am." Spouses and patients may attribute different meanings to other aspects of their experience as well. For example, when seeing their loved one in pain, many spouses felt helpless and fearful. Once the pain was controlled, they felt peaceful and relaxed and interpreted this as an indication that the couple would return to their old routines. The meaning attributed to the patient's experience also influences spousal bereavement. For example, spouses who witnessed distressing sights and sounds as the patient was dying experienced posttraumatic stress and much distress after the death.[31]

Children tended to reflect on and reevaluate all aspects of their lives: "It puts in perspective how important some of our goals are. . . . Having financial independence and being able to retire at a decent age. . . . Those things are important, but not at the expense of sacrificing today."

Living Day to Day

Not all families reached the point of living day to day. If patients were able to find some meaning in their experience, then they were better able to adopt an attitude of living each day. Their attitude was characterized by "making the most of it." As one patient described it, "There's not much point in going over things in the past; not much point in projecting yourself too far into the future either. It's the current time that counts." Patients who were unable to find much meaning in their experience, or who didn't search for meaning, focused more on "getting through it." As Ralph said with determination, "Sure, I am getting weaker. I know I am sick. . . . But I will get through this!"

Spouses who searched for meaning focused on "making the best of it" while making every effort to enjoy the time they had left with their partner. Other spouses simply endured the situation without paying much attention to philosophizing about the experience. Children often had difficulty concentrating on living day to day, because they were unable to defer their obligations and therefore were constantly worrying about what else needed to be done. However, some children were still able to convey an attitude of "Live for today, today—worry about tomorrow, tomorrow."

Preparing for Death

Preparing for death involved concrete actions that would have benefit in the future, after the patient died. Patients had their family's needs uppermost in their minds and worked hard to teach or guide family members with regard to various tasks and activities that the patient would no longer be around to do. Patients were committed to leaving legacies for their loved ones, not only as a means of being remembered but also as a way of comforting loved ones in their grief. Joe spent time "jotting down a few Mr. Fix-it pointers" for his wife and son. Ralph's energy was consumed by focusing on the work he still had to do, so he was unable to consider what he might do for his wife and daughter.

Spouses concentrated on meeting the patient's wishes. Whatever the patient wanted, spouses would try to do. They attended to practical details and anticipated their future in practical ways. Children offered considerable help to their parents with legal and financial matters. They also prepared their own children for what was to come. A central aspect was reassuring the dying parent that they would take care of the surviving parent. Children also prepared for the death by envisioning their future without their parent: "I think about it sometimes . . . about how my children will never have a grandfather. It makes me so sad. That's why the photos we have been taking are so important to me. . . . They will show our children who their grandfather was."

Palliative Care for Diagnoses Other Than Cancer

Traditionally, palliative care practice and discussions have focused on families of cancer patients, while care of the patient with cardiac disease has traditionally focused on restoring health and enabling a return to normal life. For most patients with heart disease, and particularly for those with heart failure, the decline in functional status is slower than for patients diagnosed with cancer.[21] However, if palliative care is considered only after disease-related care fails or becomes too burdensome, the opportunity for patients to achieve symptom relief, and for patients and family members to engage in the positive and conscious process of fading away, may be lost. Following a model of care where issues of treatment and end-of-life care are discussed early and throughout the illness trajectory facilitates patient and family coping and enables nurses to optimally support families.

Varying disease trajectories for other conditions,[32,33] including dementia, also influence the nature of support that nurses provide patients and families. For example, the support needed by families of patients with dementia often occurs before the life-limiting nature of the condition is recognized by families. In dementia care, there may be significantly more need than with other illnesses to form support groups for families, offer respite care, educate families, and try to relieve families' feelings of guilt.[34]

Family Involvement According to Location of Care

Over the past century, nursing homes and hospitals increasingly have become the site of death. A landmark national study evaluated the US dying experience at home and in institutional settings.[35] Family members of 1578 deceased individuals were asked via telephone survey about the patient's experience at the last place of care at which the patient spent >48 hours. Results showed that two-thirds (67.2%) of patients were last cared for in an institution; little has changed in the intervening years. Family members reported greater satisfaction with patient's symptom management, and with emotional support for both the patient and family, if they received care at home with hospice services. Families have greater opportunities for involvement in the care if home care is possible. Family involvement in hospital care also makes for better outcomes.[36] Nurses, therefore, must consider how best to include families in the care of their dying loved ones, regardless of the location of care.

Large variations exist in the provision of home-based palliative and terminal care across the United States, although the development of hospice home services has enabled increasing numbers of seriously ill patients to experience care at home. However, dying at home can present special challenges for family members.[37] Lack of support and lack of confidence have been found to be determinants contributing to hospital admissions and the breakdown of informal caregiving for people with a life-threatening illness. A lack of support from the healthcare system is given as the reason many caregivers have to admit their loved one to the hospital.[12] They also report that fragmentation of services and lack of forward planning jeopardizes the success of home care.[12]

> **Box 3.1 Family Members' Decisions to Care for Someone at Home Are Influenced by Three Major Factors**
>
> 1. Making promises to care for the loved one at home,
> 2. The desire to maintain as much as possible a "normal" life for the patient and themselves, and
> 3. Negative experiences with institutional care.

The decision to care for a family member at home has a profound effect on family members (Box 3.1).[15,16] Many caregivers believe that providing home care for their loved one is the only option.[12] Some make uninformed decisions, giving little consideration to the implications of their decision. Such decisions are often made early in the patient's disease trajectory or when the patient was imminently dying. The patient's needs and wishes often drive decisions, with caregivers paying little attention to their own needs.[12] Negotiated decisions for home care typically occur if caregivers and patients are able to talk openly about dying, and have done so throughout the disease trajectory. For some families, a home death brings additional burdens, worries, and responsibilities.[37]

Family members may be reluctant to ask for help or to let their needs be known. They tend not to think of themselves as the target of professional interventions. When working with caregiving families, healthcare providers can facilitate the sharing of perspectives, to allow for decisions that would work well for all concerned. Ideally, such discussions begin early in the disease trajectory. It is important that attention is paid to improving hospital end-of-life care so that families feel they have a meaningful alternative to home care. There is an emotional impact in providing palliative care at home. The task caregiving imposes on family caregivers may seem overwhelming at times. Care must be provided within the framework of an interdisciplinary team[38] so that families can benefit from a whole set of services needed to support death at home.

Some simple guidelines for families can serve to encourage their coping. For example, caregivers should be told to keep a small notebook handy for jotting down questions and answers. They should be advised to have the notebook with them whenever they talk with a member of the palliative care team. Family members should be reassured that nothing is trivial. All questions are important, and all observations are valuable. They should be encouraged to say when they do not understand something, and to ask for information to be repeated as necessary. They should reassure family members that asking for help is not a sign of failure, but rather a sign of good common sense. Following such simple guidelines helps keep families from feeling overwhelmed. And, if they do feel "out of control," such guidelines, simple as they may seem, give family members some concrete action they can take to help with whatever the situation may be.

Caregiving at a Distance

About 89% of all informal caregivers are related to the care recipient,[39] but not all caregiving is provided by family members who live with, or are geographically close to, the patient. Distant caregiving, the provision of instrumental and/or emotional support to an ill loved one who lives a long distance from the caregiver, is prevalent in today's changing society.

Adult children often live far from their parents and find themselves caregiving from a distance. Millions of Americans are distant caregivers, and the number is only expected to increase as baby boomers and their parents age.[40] An estimated 15% of caregivers live an hour or more from their loved one.[39] These adult children are dealing with the added challenges and stressors associated with living at a distance, such as lack of nearby family support. There is some indication that stress related to the distant caregiving is quite common in caregivers[41]; otherwise, little is known about their experiences. Most interventions have been designed to support local caregivers. Interventions to decrease caregiver burden and improve caregiver well-being may not be as applicable to distant caregivers, who may need extra flexibility and accommodations, such as increased telephone communication, in order to meet their needs.

Advance Care Planning

Whether care is provided in hospital or by families in the home or at a distance, patients at the end of life may not be able to make decisions about their own care. Family members, therefore, are often asked to make those decisions on the patient's behalf, yet they may not know explicitly what the patient would want. Advance care planning is a process that allows the patient's preferences to be made known to the family and to healthcare professionals. It involves discussions between the patient and his or her family and friends, as well as written instructions in the event that a patient can no longer express his or her choices verbally. Advance care planning is best begun while family members are healthy but when someone is ill, then as early as possible in the illness experience and revisited as needed because preferences can change over time.[42,43]

However, even in the less than 30% of cases when an adult has an advance directive, it may be neither specific enough nor available when needed.[44] Clinicians should ask whether advance directives are available, and they might invite family discussion regardless of whether or not such directives are in place. It is important for clinicians to be familiar with a patient's advance directive and to advocate for the patient if needed. Information about advance directives is available from the American Cancer Society.[45]

Guidelines for Nursing Interventions

Despite differences across and between cultures, similarities exist in regard to basic needs for support, dignity, and connections with others.[46–49] Much of the nursing literature, which provides guidelines for nursing care, addresses the importance of four major interventions that have relevance for all members of the palliative care team:

1. *Maintain hope* in patients and their family members. As families pass through the illness trajectory, the nature of their hope changes from hope for cure, to hope for remission, to hope for comfort, to hope for a good death. Offering hope during fading away can be as simple as reassuring families that everything will be done to ensure the patient's comfort. Talking about the past also can help some families by reaffirming the good times spent together and the ongoing connections that will continue among family members. Referring to the future beyond the immediate suffering and emotional pain can also sustain hope. For example, when adult children reassure the ill parent that they will care for the other parent, the patient is hopeful that the surviving spouse will be all right.

2. *Involve families* in all aspects of care. Include them in decision-making, and encourage active participation in the physical care of the patient. This is their life—they have the right to control it as they will. Involvement is especially important for children when a family member is very ill. The more children are involved in care during the terminal phase, and in the activities that follow the death, the better able they are to cope with bereavement.[50,51]

3. *Offer information.* Tell families about what is happening in straightforward terms and about what they can expect to happen, particularly about the patient's condition and the process their loved one is to undergo. Doing so also provides families with a sense of control. Initiate the discussion of relevant issues that family members themselves may hesitate to mention. For example, the nurse might say, "Many family members feel as if they are being pulled in two or more directions when a loved one is very ill. They want to spend as much time as possible with the patient, but they also feel the pull of their own daily lives, careers, or families. How does this fit with your experience?"

4. *Communicate openly.* Open and honest communication with nurses and other health professionals is frequently the most important need of families. They need to be informed; they need opportunities to ask questions and to have their questions answered in terms that they can comprehend. Open communication among team members is basic to open communication with the families.

These four broad interventions assist healthcare providers in providing good palliative care; the following guidelines offer further direction (Tables 3.1 and 3.2). They are derived from the direct accounts of patients, spouses, and children about the strategies they used to cope with the dimensions of fading away.

Table 3.1 Dimensions of Family Functioning: Examples of the Range of Behaviors

More Helpful	Less Helpful
Integrating the Past	
Describe the painful experiences as they relate to present experience	Describe past experiences repeatedly
Describe positive and negative feelings concerning the past	Dwell on painful feelings associated with past experiences
Incorporate learning from the past into subsequent experiences	Do not integrate learning from the past to the current situation
Reminisce about pleasurable experiences in the past	Focus on trying to "fix" the past to create happy memories that are absent from their family life
Dealing With Feelings	
Express a range of feelings including vulnerability, fear, and uncertainty	Express predominantly negative feelings, such as anger, hurt, bitterness, and fear
Acknowledge paradoxical feelings	Acknowledge little uncertainty or few paradoxical feelings
Solving Problems	
Identify problems as they occur	Focus more on fault finding than on finding solutions
Reach consensus about a problem and possible courses of action	Dwell on the emotions associated with the problem
Consider multiple options	Unable to clearly communicate needs and expectations
Open to suggestions	Feel powerless about influencing the care they are receiving
Approach problems as a team rather than as individuals	Display exaggerated response to unexpected events
	Withhold information from or inaccurately share information with other family members
Utilizing Resources	
Utilize a wide range of resources	Utilize few resources
Open to accepting support	Reluctant to seek help or accept offers of help
Open to suggestions regarding resources	Receive help mostly from formal sources rather than from informal support networks
Take the initiative in procuring additional resources	Avoid seeking or exploring additional resources on their own
Express satisfaction with results obtained	Express dissatisfaction with help received
Describe the involvement of many friends, acquaintances, and support persons	Describe fewer friends and acquaintances who offer help
Considering Others	
Acknowledge multidimensional effects of situation on other family members	Focus concern on own emotional needs

(continued)

Table 3.1 (Continued)

More Helpful	Less Helpful
Express concern for well-being of other family members	Fail to acknowledge or minimize extra tasks taken on by others
Focus concern on patient's well-being	Focus on own self
Appreciate individualized attention from healthcare professionals, but do not express strong need for such attention	Display inordinate need for individualized attention
Direct concerns about how other family members are managing rather than about themselves	Focus concerns on themselves
Identify characteristic coping styles of family unit and of individual members	Describe own characteristic coping styles rather than the characteristic way the family as a unit coped
Demonstrate warmth and caring toward other family members	Allow one member to dominate group interaction
Consider present situation as potential opportunity for family's growth and development	Lack comfort with expressing true feelings in the family group
Value contributions of all family members	Feign group consensus where none exists
Describe a history of closeness among family members	Describe few family interactions prior to illness
Fulfilling Roles	
Demonstrate flexibility in adapting to role changes	Demonstrate rigidity in adapting to role changes and responsibilities
Share extra responsibilities willingly	Demonstrate less sharing of responsibilities created by extra demands of patient care
Adjust priorities to incorporate extra demands of patient care and express satisfaction with this decision	Refer to caregiving as a duty or obligation
Enlist assistance as needed and entrust responsibilities to others	Criticize or mistrust caregiving provided by others
Tolerating Differences	
Allow differing opinions and beliefs within the family	Display intolerance for differing opinions or approaches of caregiving
Tolerate different views from people outside the family	Demonstrate critical views of friends who fail to respond as expected
Willing to examine own belief and value systems	Adhere rigidly to belief and value systems
From reference 52.	

Table 3.2 Family Functioning: Guidelines for Interventions in Palliative Care

Assessing Family Functioning	Solving Problems
Use dimensions of family functioning to assess families. For example: Do members focus their concern on the patient's well-being and recognize the effect of the situation on other family members, or do family members focus their concerns on their own individual needs and minimize how others might be affected? Putting your assessment of all the dimensions together will help you determine to what degree you are dealing with a more cohesive family unit or a more loosely coupled group of individuals, and hence what approaches are most appropriate.	*Use your assessment of family functioning to guide your approaches.* For example, in families where there is little consensus about the problems, rigidity in beliefs, and inflexibility in roles and relationships, the common rule of thumb—offering families various options so they may choose those that suit them best—tends to be less successful. For these families, carefully consider which resource provides the best possible fit for that particular family. Offer resources slowly, perhaps one at a time. Focus considerable attention on the degree of disruption associated with the introduction of the resource, and prepare the family for the change that ensues. Otherwise, the family may reject the resource as unsuitable and perceive the experience as yet another example of failure of the healthcare system to meet their needs.
Be prepared to collect information over time and from different family members. Some family members may not be willing to reveal their true feelings until they have developed trust. Others may be reluctant to share differing viewpoints in the presence of one another. In some families, certain individuals take on the role of spokesperson for the family. Assessing whether everyone in the family shares the viewpoints of the spokesperson, or whether different family members have divergent opinions but are reluctant to share them, is a critical part of the assessment.	*Be aware of the limitations of family conferences and be prepared to follow up.* Family conferences work well for more cohesive family units. However, where more disparity exists among the members, they may not follow through with the decisions made, even though consensus was apparently achieved. Though not voicing their disagreement, some family members may not be committed to the solution put forward and may disregard the agreed-on plan. The nurse needs to follow up to ensure that any trouble spots are addressed.
Listen to the family's story and use clinical judgment to determine where intervention is required. Part of understanding a family is listening to their story. In some families, the stories tend to be repeated and the feelings associated with them resurface. Talking about the past is a way of being for some families. It is important that the nurse determine whether family members are repeatedly telling their story because they want to be better understood or because they want help to change the way their family deals with the situation. Most often the stories are retold simply because family members want the nurse to understand them and their situation better, not because they are looking for help to change the way their family functions.	*Be prepared to repeat information.* In less cohesive families, do not assume that information will be accurately and openly shared with other family members. You may have to repeat information several times to different family members and repeat answers to the same questions from various family members.

(continued)

Table 3.2 (Continued)

Assessing Family Functioning	Solving Problems
	Evaluate the appropriateness of support groups. Support groups can be a valuable resource. They help by providing people with the opportunity to hear the perspectives of others in similar situations. However, some family members need more individualized attention than a support group provides. They do not benefit from hearing how others have experienced the situation and dealt with the problems. They need one-to-one interaction focused on themselves with someone with whom they have developed trust.
	Adjust care to the level of family functioning. Some families are more overwhelmed by the palliative care experience than others. Understanding family functioning can help nurses appreciate that expectations for some families to "pull together" to cope with the stress of palliative care may be unrealistic. Nurses need to adjust their care according to the family's way of functioning and be prepared for the fact that working with some families is more demanding and the outcomes achieved are less optimal.

From Davies B, Chekryn Reimer J, Brown P, Martens N. Fading Away: The Experience of Transition in Families With Terminal Illness. Amityville, NY: Baywood; 1995.

Summary

Family-centered care is a basic tenet of palliative care. Illness is incorporated into every aspect of family life. The patient's illness affects the whole family, and in turn the family's responses affect the patient. Supporting families in palliative care means that nurses must plan their care with an understanding not only of the individual patient's needs but also of the family system within which the patient functions.

References

1. US Census Bureau. America's families and living arrangements: 2011. Family status and household relationship of people 15 years and over, by marital status, age, and sex: 2011 (Table A2). Retrieved from http://www.census.gov/population/www/socdemo/hh-fam/cps2011.html.

2. Panke JT, Ferrell BR. The family perspective. In: Hanks G, Cherny N, Christakis NA, Fallon M, Kaasa S, Portenoy RK, eds. Oxford Textbook of Palliative Medicine. 4th ed. Oxford: Oxford University Press; 2010:1437–1444.

3. Field MJ, Cassell CK, eds. Approaching Death: Improving Care at the End of Life. Washington, DC: National Academy Press, 1997.

4. Wittenberg-Lyles E, Demiris G, Oliver DP, Burt S. Reciprocal suffering: caregiver concerns during hospice care. J Pain Symptom Manage. 2011;41(2):383–393.

5. Northouse LL, Katapodi MC, Song L, Zhang L, Mood DW. Interventions with family caregivers of cancer patients: Meta-analysis of randomized trials. CA: Cancer J Clin. 2010;60:317–339.

6. Stajduhar KI, Martin WL, Barwich D, Fyles G. Factors influencing family caregivers' ability to cope with providing end-of-life cancer care at home. Canc Nurs. 2008;31:77–85.

7. Aoun S, McGonigley R, Abernethy A, Currow DC. Caregivers of people with neurodegenerative diseases: profile and unmet needs from a population-based survey in South Australia. J Pall Med. 2010;13(6):653–661.

8. Milberg A, Olsson EC, Jakobsson M, Olsson M, Friedrichsen M. Family members' perceived needs for bereavement follow-up. J Pain Symptom Manage. 2008;35(1):58–69.

9. Milberg A, Strang P. Protection against perceptions of powerlessness and helplessness during palliative care: the family members' perspective. Pall Supp Care. 2011;9(3):251–262.

10. Corà A, Partinico M, Munafò M, Palomba D. Health risk factors in caregivers of terminal cancer patients: a pilot study. Cancer Nurs. 2012;35(1):38–47.

11. Kenny P, Hall J, Zapart S, Davis PR. Informal care and home-based palliative care: the health-related quality of life of carers. J Pain Symptom Manage. 2010;40(1):35–48.

12. Robinson CA, Pesut B, Bottorff JL. Supporting rural family palliative caregivers. J Fam Nurs. 2012;18(4):467–490.

13. Funk L, Stajduhar KI, Toye C, Aoun S, Grande GE, Todd CJ. Part 2: Home-based family caregiving at the end of life: a

comprehensive review of published qualitative research (1998–2008). Pall Med. 2010;24(6):507–607.

14. Grande G, Stajduhar K, Aoun S, et al. Supporting lay carers in end of life care: current gaps and future priorities. Pall Med. 2009;23(4):339–344.

15. Stajduhar K, Funk L, Jakobsson E, Ohlen J. A critical analysis of health promotion and "empowerment" in the context of palliative family care-giving. Nurs Inquiry. 2010;17(3):221–230.

16. Stajduhar K, Funk L, Toye C, Grande GE, Soun S, Todd CJ. Part 1: Home based family caregiving at the end of life: a comprehensive review of published quantitative research (1998–2008). Pall Med. 2010;24(6):573–593.

17. Benzein EG, Saveman B. Health-promoting conversations about hope and suffering with couples in palliative care. Int J Palliat Nurse. 2008;14:439–445.

18. Fine E, Reid MC, Shengelia R, Adelman RD. Directly observed patient–physician discussions in palliative and end-of-life care: a systematic review of the literature. J Palliat Med. 2010;13(5):595–603.

19. Rhodes RL, Mitchell SL, Miller SC, Connor SR, Teno JM. Bereaved family members' evaluation of hospice care: what factors influence overall satisfaction with care? J Pain Sympt Manage. 2008;35:365–371.

20. Hasson F, Kernohan WG, McLaughlin M, et al. An exploration into the palliative and end-of-life experiences of carers of people with Parkinson's disease. Palliat Med. 2010;24(7):731–736.

21. Saunders MM. Factors associated with caregiver burden in heart failure family caregivers. West J Nurs Res. 2008;30(8):943–959.

22. Aoun SM, Connors SL, Priddis L, Breen LJ, Colyer S. Motor neurone disease family carers' experiences of caring, palliative care and bereavement: an exploratory qualitative study. Palliat Med. 2012;26(6):842–850.

23. Hennings J, Froggatt K, Keady J. Approaching the end of life and dying with dementia in care homes: the accounts of family carers. Rev Clin Geront. 2010;20:114–127.

24. World Health Organization. Palliative Care for Older People: Better Practices. Author 2011. Retrieved from http://www.euro.who.int/__data/assets/pdf_file/0017/143153/e95052.pdf.

25. Davies B, Chekryn Reimer J, Brown P, Martens N. Fading Away: The Experience of Transition in Families With Terminal Illness. Amityville, NY: Baywood; 1995.

26. Bridges W. Transitions: Making Sense of Life's Changes. Reading, MA: Addison-Wesley; 1980.

27. Stajduhar KI, Martin WL, Barwich D, Fyles G. Factors influencing family caregivers' ability to cope with providing end-of-life cancer care at home. Cancer Nurs. 2008;31(1):77–85.

28. Fitzsimons D, Mullan D, Wilson JS, et al. The challenge of patients' unmet palliative care needs in the final stages of chronic illness. Palliat Med. 2007;21(4):313–322.

29. Wolkowski A, Carr SM, Clarke CL. What does respite care mean for palliative care service users and carers? Messages from a conceptual mapping. Int J Palliat Nurs. 2010;16(8):388–392.

30. Hexem KR, Mollen CJ, Carroll K, Lanctot DA, Feudtner C. How parents of children receiving pediatric palliative care use religion, spirituality, or life philosophy in tough times. J Palliat Med. 2011;14(1):39–44.

31. Sanderson C, Lobb EA, Mowll J, Butow PN, McGowan N, Price MA. Signs of post-traumatic stress disorder in caregivers following an expected death: a qualitative study. Palliat Med. 2013;27(7):625–631.

32. Murray SA, Kendall M, Boyd K, Sheikh A. Illness trajectories and palliative care. BMJ. 2005;330(7498):1007–1011.

33. Murray SA, Sheikh A. Care for all at the end of life. BMJ. 2008;336(7650):958–959.

34. van der Steen JT, Radbruch L, Hertogh CMPM, et al. White paper defining optimal palliative care in older people with dementia: a Delphi study and recommendations from the European Association for Palliative Care. Palliat Med. July 2013; published online before print.

35. Teno JM, Clarridge BR, Casey V, et al. Family perspectives on end-of-life care at the last place of death. JAMA. 2004;291:88–93.

36. Spichiger E. Family experiences of hospital end-of-life care in Switzerland: an interpretive phenomenological study. Int J Palliat Nurs. 2009;15(7):332–337.

37. Stajduhar K. Burdens of family caregiving at the end of life. Clin Invest Med. 2013;36(3):E121–E126.

38. Klarare A, Hagelin CL, Fürst CJ, Fossum B. Team interactions in specialized palliative care teams: a qualitative study. J Palliat Med. 2013;16(9):1062–1069.

39. National Alliance for Caregiving; in collaboration with AARP. Caregiving in the U.S.: A Focused Look at Those Caring for the 50+. Author; 2009. Retrieved from http://assets.aarp.org/rgcenter/il/caregiving_09.pdf.

40. National Institute on Aging. So Far Away: 20 Questions and Answers About Long-Distance Caregiving. NIH Publication No. 10-5496. Bethseda MD: National Institutes of Health, 2011. Retrieved from http://www.nia.nih.gov/sites/default/files/so_far_away_twenty_questions_about_long-distance_caregiving.pdf.

41. Alzheimer's Association. Alzheimer's Disease: Facts and Figures. Author; 2013. Retrieved from http://www.alz.org/alzheimers_disease_facts_and_figures.asp.

42. Robinson CA. Advance care planning: re-visioning our ethical approach. Can J Nurs Res. 2011;43(2):18–37.

43. Robinson CA. "Our best hope is a cure": hope in the context of advance care planning. Pall Supp Care. 2012;10:75–82.

44. Dunn PM, Tolle SW, Moss AH, Black JS. The POLST paradigm: respecting the wishes of patients and families. Ann Long-Term Care. 2007;15(9):33–40.

45. American Cancer Society. Advance Directives. Author; 2011. Retrieved from http://www.cancer.org/acs/groups/cid/documents/webcontent/002016-pdf.pdf.

46. Yeh P-M, Bull M. Influences of spiritual well-being and coping on mental health of family caregivers for elders. Res Gerontol Nurs. 2009;2(3):173–181.

47 Ferrell B, Otis-Green S, Economou D. Spirituality in cancer care at the end of life. Cancer J. 2013;19(5):431–437.

48. Donovan R, Williams A, Stajduhar K, Brazil K, Marshall D. The influence of culture on home-based family caregiving at end-of-life: a case study of Dutch reformed family care givers in Ontario, Canada. Soc Sci Med. 2011;72(3):338–346.

49. Kongsuwan W, Chaipetch O, Matchim Y. Thai Buddhist families' perspective of a peaceful death. Nurs Crit Care. 2012;17(3):151–159.

50. Davies B. Environmental factors affecting sibling bereavement. In: Davies B. Shadows in the Sun: Experiences of Sibling Bereavement in Childhood. Philadelphia: Brunner/Mazel; 1999:123–148.

51. Steele R, Robinson C, Hansen L, Widger, K. Families and palliative/end-of-life care. In Kaakinen J, Gedalfy-Duff V, Coehlo D, Hanson S, eds. Family Health Care Nursing: Theory, Practice and Research. 4th ed. Philadelphia: F. A. Davis; 2010:273–306.

52. Davies B, Reimer J, Martens N. Family functioning and its implications for palliative care. J Palliat Care. 1994;10:35–36.

Chapter 4

Planning for the Actual Death

Patricia Berry and Julie Griffie

The central theme of this chapter is that care of the family is central to care of the dying. While the physiology of dying is often the same for most expected deaths, the psychological, spiritual, cultural, and family issues are as unique and varied as the patients and families themselves. As death nears, the goals of care need to be discussed and appropriately redefined. Some treatments may be discontinued, and symptoms may intensify, subside, or appear anew. Physiological changes as death approaches should be normalized, explained, and interpreted to the patient whenever possible, as well as to the family and caregivers. The nurse occupies a key position in assisting patients' family members at the time of death, supporting and/ or suggesting death rituals, caring for the body after death, and facilitating early grief work. This chapter discusses some key issues surrounding the death itself, including advance planning, evolving and changing choices and goals of care, the changing focus of care as death nears, common signs and symptoms of nearing death and their management, and care of the patient and family at time of death. It concludes with two case examples illustrating the chapter's content.

Key Points

- It is the nurse who provides much of the care and support to patients and families throughout the disease trajectory and the one who is most likely to be present at the time of death.
- With this comes a special responsibility for the nurse to acquire the necessary clinical knowledge and interpersonal skills to provide care to the patient and family as life draws to a close.
- Assessment and management of symptoms remain a priority especially as death approaches.
- Care of the body after death, honoring rituals and individual requests is critically important in communicating to the family that the person who died was important and valued.

Case Study: Jim With Stage III Lung Cancer

I had known Jim from my church and community for almost half of my lifetime. We met when we were both newly married and just starting down the road of life. He was brilliant, a shining star in the crowd. With a loving wife of 30+ years, he had nurtured many students, but never had the joy of being a biological father. Instead, he nurtured everyone around him. About three years ago, he suddenly appeared in our clinic. Suddenly, he was "our patient," with Stage III lung cancer. He analyzed and plotted out each step of his treatment plan, and was able to successfully stay "on top" of (control) his cancer for 2 years.

When headaches started, he had a positive neurological workup, was scanned and started on radiation therapy along with a different chemotherapy. And then, one bright Monday morning, his wife arrived to tell us that Jim had experienced a seizure, and had been admitted through the ER the previous night. A neurooncologist had seen him and there was a plan for placement of an Ommaya reservoir. We had all walked this path before with other patients, and were in need of a plan for how we would assure that both our friend and his wife truly understood risks and benefits of these next steps. No one wanted to see Jim not be able to "be Jim." It was time for us to seriously nurture Jim and his wife more aggressively, as we helped them prepare for Jim's death.

Where Death Occurs

Terminally ill persons are cared for in a variety of settings, including home settings with hospice care or traditional home care, hospice residential facilities, nursing homes, assisted living facilities, hospitals, intensive care units, prisons, and group homes. Deaths in intensive care settings may present special challenges, such as restrictive visiting hours and lack of space and less privacy for families—shortcomings that can be addressed by thoughtful and creative nursing care. Likewise, death in a nursing home setting may also offer unique challenges. Regardless of the setting, anticipating and managing pain and symptoms can minimize distress and maximize quality of life. Families can be supported in a way that optimizes use of valuable time and lessens distress during the bereavement period.

The Importance of Family as Death Draws Near

The patient's family is especially important as death nears. Family members may become full- or part-time caregivers; daughters and sons may find themselves in a position to "parent" their parents; and family issues, long forgotten or ignored, may surface. Although "family" is often thought of in traditional terms, a family may take on several forms and configurations. For the purposes of this chapter, the definition of family recognizes that many patients have nontraditional families and may be cared for by a large extended entity, such as a church community, a group of supportive friends, or the staff of a healthcare facility. Family is defined broadly to include not only persons bound by biology or legal ties but also those whom the patient defines or who define themselves as "close others" or who function for the patient as a family member would, including nurturance, intimacy, and economic, social, and psychological support in times of need; support in illness (including dealing with those outside the family); and companionship.

Symptoms at End of Life

There is a constellation of symptoms common throughout the course of end-stage disease, and symptoms that appear during the period immediately preceding death, most often 2–3 days prior. It is estimated that up to 52% of patients have refractory symptoms at the very end of life that at times require palliative sedation.[1] In a recent systematic review of signs of impending death and symptoms in the last 2 weeks of life, a total of 43 unique symptoms were identified, with dyspnea (56.7%), pain (52.4%), noisy breathing/respiratory congestion (51.4%), and confusion (50.1%) as the most common.[2] Within a few days of death, many patients experience a higher frequency of noisy and moist breathing, urinary incontinence and retention, restlessness, agitation, delirium, and nausea and vomiting.[3–5] Symptoms that occur with less frequency include sweating and myoclonus, with myoclonus sometimes occurring as a reversible toxic effect of morphine, especially in older patients and those with renal impairment.[2,6] In most studies, symptoms requiring maximum diligence in assessment, prevention, and aggressive treatment during the final day or two before death are respiratory tract secretions/moist breathing, pain, dyspnea, and agitated delirium, which is very common.[2,7–8] For some patients, the pathway to death is characterized by progressive sleepiness leading to coma and death. For others, the pathway to death is marked by increasing symptoms, including restlessness, confusion, hallucinations, sometimes seizure activity, and then coma and death.[9] Assessment and intervention is focused on identifying those persons who are on the more difficult pathway and aggressively treating their symptoms to assure a peaceful death. Persons with cognitive impairment and the inability to self-report or communicate require specific attention to symptoms, especially as death nears. The nurse plays a key role in assessing and anticipating symptoms, acting promptly to assure, if at all possible, that symptoms are aggressively prevented and managed before they become severe. The nurse also has an important role in educating family members and other caregivers about the assessment, treatment, and ongoing evaluation of these symptoms.

Patient Dependency and Nursing Impact as Death Approaches

Patients experience profound dependency as death becomes close. Families are frequently called on to assume total caregiving duties, disrupting their own responsibilities for home, children, and career. Patients and families experience this time through the unique lens of their own perspective and form their own unique meaning. Carl Rogers's theory of helping relationships suggests that the characteristics of a helping relationship are empathy, unconditional positive regard, and genuineness.[10] These characteristics are part of the nurse's approach to patients and families when facilitating care at the end of life. In addition, "attention to detail" is crucial to providing patient-and family-centered quality palliative care.[11–12]

Foundation for Facilitating and Providing Supportive Relationships

- Empathy: the ability to put oneself in the other person's place, trying to understand the patient or client from his or her own frame of reference; it also requires the deliberate setting aside of one's own frame of reference and bias.

- Unconditional positive regard: a warm feeling toward others, with a non-judgmental acceptance of all they reveal themselves to be; the ability to convey a sense of respect and esteem at a time and place in which it is particularly important to do so.

- Genuineness: the ability to convey trustworthiness and openness that is real rather than a professional facade; also the ability to admit that one has limitations, makes mistakes, and does not have all the answers.

- Attention to detail: the learned and practiced ability to think critically about a situation and not make assumptions. The nurse, for example, discusses challenging patient and family concerns with colleagues and other members of the interdisciplinary team. The nurse considers every "what if" before making a decision and, in particular, before making any judgment. Finally, the nurse is constantly aware of how his or her actions, attitudes, and words may be interpreted—or misinterpreted— by others.

The events and interactions at the bedside of a dying person set the tone for the patient's care and form lasting memories for family members. The time of death and the care received by both the individual who has died and the family members who are present are predominant aspects of the survivors' memories of this event.

The Process

Making sure that the patient's values, beliefs, and goals of care direct the care that they receive, and that they or their healthcare agent have the necessary information to make informed choices, is an important nursing role. Effective communication allows the nurse to guide the patient and family through what may seem like a myriad of choices and endless decisions to be made. Advance care planning is a key part of this process.

Advance Planning: Evolving Choices and Goals of Care

Healthcare choices related to wellness are generally viewed as clear-cut or easy. We have an infection, we seek treatment, and the treatment choices are obvious. As wellness moves along the healthcare continuum to illness, choices become less clear and consequences of choices have a significantly greater impact. Many end-of-life illnesses manifest with well-known and well-documented natural courses. Providing the patient and family with information on the natural course of the disease at appropriate intervals is a critical function of healthcare providers such as nurses. Providing an opening for discussion, such as, "Would you like to talk about the future?" "Do you have any concerns that I can help you address?" or "It seems you are not as active as you were before," may allow a much-needed discussion of fears and concerns about impending death. Family members may request information that patients do not wish to know. With the patient's permission, discussions with the family may occur in the patient's absence. Family members may also need coaching to initiate end-of-life discussions with the patient. End-of-life goal setting is greatly enhanced when the patient is aware of the support of family. The patient who is capable of participating in and making decisions is always the acknowledged decision maker. The involvement of family ensures maximal consensus for patient support as decisions are actually implemented. Decisions for patients who lack decision-making capacity should be made by a consensus approach, using family conference methodology. If documents such as a durable power of attorney for healthcare or a living will are available, they can be used as a guide for examining wishes that influence decision-making and goal setting. The decision maker, usually the person named as healthcare power of attorney (HCPOA), or the patient's primary family members, should be clearly identified.

To facilitate decision-making, convening a family conference that involves the decision makers (decisional patient, family members, and the HCPOA), the patient's physician or provider, nurse, chaplain, and social worker is ideal. A history of how the patient's healthcare status evolved from diagnosis to the present is reviewed. The family is presented with the natural course of the disease. Choices on how care may proceed, including prognostic estimations and the benefits and burdens of treatments are reviewed. Guidance or support for those choices is provided based on existing data and clinical experience with the particular disease in relation to the current status of the patient. If no consensus for the needed decisions occurs, decision-making is postponed. Third-party support by a trusted individual or consultant may then be enlisted. Decisions by patients and families cross the spectrum of care ranging from continuing treatment for the actual disease, such as undergoing chemotherapy or renal dialysis or utilization of medications, to initiating cardiopulmonary resuscitation (CPR). The healthcare provider works with the patient and family, making care decisions for specific treatments and timing treatment discontinuance within a clear and logical framework.

A goal-setting discussion may determine a patient's personal framework for care, such as:

- Treatment and enrollment in any clinical studies for which I am eligible.
- Treatment as long as statistically there is a greater than 50% chance of response.
- Full treatment as long as I am ambulatory and able to come to the clinic or office.

- Treatment only of "fixable" conditions such as infections or blood glucose levels.
- Treatment only for controlling symptomatic aspects of disease.

Once a "goals of care" framework has been established with the patient, the appropriateness of interventions such as CPR, renal dialysis, or intravenous antibiotics is clear. For instance, if the patient states a desire for renal dialysis as long as transportation to the clinic is possible without the use of an ambulance, the endpoint of dialysis treatment is quite clear. At this point, the futility of CPR would also be apparent. Allowing a patient to determine when the treatment is a burden that is unjustified by his or her value system, and communicating this determination to family and caregivers, is perhaps the most pivotal point in management of the patient's care (Box 4.1).

Changing the Focus of Care as Death Nears

As death nears, the rhythm of care changes; visiting hours in an institutional setting are relaxed, the routines of care, for example taking vital signs, tracking intake and output, and daily weights become less important, and treatments automatically associated with caring for any patient are considered in the context of benefit and burden. The nurse also plays an important role in advocating on behalf of the patient, interpreting the goals of care to colleagues and assuring that the care delivered is consistent with the goals and preferences of the patient and/or family.

Vital Signs

If the plan of care no longer involves intervening in changes in blood pressure and pulse rate, the measurements should cease. The time spent taking vital signs can then be redirected to assessment of patient comfort and provision of family support. Changes in respiratory rate are visually noted and do not require routine monitoring of rates, unless symptom management issues develop that could be more accurately assessed by measurement of vital signs. The measurement of body temperature using a noninvasive route should continue on a regular basis until death, if the patient appears uncomfortable, allowing for the detection and management of fever, a frequent symptom that can cause distress and may require management.

Fever

Fever often suggests infection. As death approaches, goal setting should include a discussion of the benefits and burdens of treating an infection. Indications for treatment of infection are based on the degree of distress and patient discomfort.[14] Pharmacological management of fever includes antipyretics, including acetaminophen and nonsteroidal antiinflammatory drugs. In some cases, treatment of an infection with an antibiotic may increase patient comfort. Ice packs, alcohol baths, and cooling blankets should be used cautiously, because they often cause more distress

Box 4.1 Moderating an End-of-Life Family Conference

I. Why: Clarify goals in your own mind.

II. Where: Provide comfort, privacy, circular seating.

III. Who: Include legal decision maker/healthcare power of attorney; family members; social support; key healthcare professionals, patient if capable to participate.

IV. How:
   A. Introduction
      1. Introduce self and others.
      2. Review meeting goals: State meeting goals and specific decisions.
      3. Establish ground rules: Each person will have a chance to ask questions and express views; no interruptions; identify legal decision maker, and describe importance of supportive decision-making.
      4. If new to patient/family, spend some time getting to know the patient as a person as well as the family.
   B. Determine what the patient/family knows.
   C. Review medical status
      1. Review current status, plan, and prognosis.
      2. Ask each family member in turn for any questions about current status, plan, and prognosis.
      3. Defer discussion of decision until the next step.
      4. Respond to emotions.
   D. Family discussion with decisional patient
      1. Ask patient, "What decision(s) are you considering?"
      2. Ask each family member, "Do you have questions or concerns about the treatment plan? How can you support the patient?"
   E. Family discussion with nondecisional patient
      1. Ask each family member in turn, "What do you believe the patient would choose if he (or she) could speak for himself (or herself)?"
      2. Ask each family member, "What do you think should be done?"
      3. Leave room to let family discuss alone.
      4. If there is consensus, go to V; if no consensus, go to F.
   F. When there is no consensus:
      1. Restate goal: "What would the patient say if he or she could speak?"
      2. Use time as ally: Schedule a follow-up conference the next day.
      3. Try further discussion: "What values is your decision based on? How will the decision affect you and other family members?"
      4. Identify legal decision-maker.
      5. Identify resources: minister/priest; other physicians; ethics committee.

V. Wrap-up
   A. Summarize consensus, decisions, and plan.
   B. Caution against unexpected outcomes.

(continued)

Box 4.1 (Continued)

    C. Identify family spokesperson for ongoing communication.

    D. Document in the chart who was present, what decisions were made, follow-up plan.

    E. Approach discontinuation of treatment as an interdisciplinary team, not just as a nursing function.

    F. Continuity: Maintain contact with family and medical team; schedule follow-up meetings as needed.

VI. Family dynamics and decisions

    A. Family structure: Respect the family hierarchy whenever possible.

    B. Established patterns of family interaction will continue.

    C. Unresolved conflicts between family members may be evident.

    D. Past problems with authority figures, doctors, and hospitals affect the process; ask specifically about bad experiences in the past.

    E. Family grieving and decision-making may include

        1. Denial: False hopes.

        2. Guilt: Fear of letting go.

        3. Depression: Passivity and inability to decide; or anger and irritability.

Source: Adapted from Ambuel B, Weissman D. Fast Fact and Concept #016: Conducting a Family Conference. 2nd ed. New York, NY: Center to Advance Palliative Care; 2009. https://www.capc.org/.

than the fever itself.[14] Fever may also suggest dehydration. As with the management of fever, interventions are guided by the degree of distress and patient discomfort. The appropriateness of beginning medically administered hydration for the treatment of fever is based on individual patient assessment, the estimated prognosis, and the goals of care. Finally, fever may suggest that death is imminent as many people develop a central fever, that is, they are cool to the touch but have an increased temperature. In this case, as with all interventions as death nears, treat for patient comfort.

Cardiopulmonary Resuscitation

Developed in the 1960s as a method of restarting the heart in the event of sudden, unexpected clinical death, CPR was originally intended for circumstances in which death was unexpected or accidental. It is not indicated in situations such as terminal irreversible illness where death is not unexpected. In general, a poor outcome of CPR is predicted in patients with advanced terminal illnesses, patients with dementia, and patients with poor functional status who depend on others for meeting their basic care needs. Poor outcomes or physical problems resulting from CPR include fractured ribs, punctured lung, brain damage if anoxia has occurred for too long, and permanent unconsciousness or persistent vegetative state.[15–16] Most importantly, the use of CPR negates the possibility of a peaceful death.

Medically Administered Fluids

The issue of medically administered or artificial hydration is emotional for many patients and families because of the role that giving and consuming fluids plays in our culture. When patients are not able to take fluids, concerns frequently surface among caregivers. A decision must be made regarding the appropriate use of fluids within the context of the patient's framework of goals. Starting artificial hydration is a relatively easy task, but the decision to stop is generally much more problematic and emotionally difficult for families. Ethical, moral, and most religious viewpoints, although not all, state that there is no difference between withholding and withdrawing a treatment such as artificial hydration. It is generally less burdensome for the patient and family not to not begin artificial hydration if this decision is acceptable in light of the specific patient circumstances.[17] Most patients and families are aware that, without fluids, death will occur quickly. The literature suggests that fluids should not be routinely administered to dying patients nor automatically withheld from them. Instead, the decision should be based on careful, individual assessment of the benefit/burden ratio. Zerwekh[18] suggests the following questions when the choice to initiate or continue hydration is evaluated.

Questions to Ask When Considering Artificial Hydration

- Is the patient's well-being likely to be enhanced by the overall effect of hydration?
- Which current symptoms are being relieved by medically administered hydration?
- Are other end-of-life symptoms being aggravated by the fluids?
- Does hydration improve the patient's level of consciousness? If so, is this within the patient's goals and wishes for end-of-life care?
- Does hydration appear to prolong the patient's survival? If so, is this within the patient's goals and wishes for end-of-life care?
- What is the effect of the infusion technology on the patient's well-being, mobility, and ability to interact and be with family?
- What is the burden of the infusion technology on the family in terms of caregiver stress, finance? Is it justified by benefit to the patient?

Research suggests that although some dying patients may benefit from dehydration, others may experience increased metabolite toxicity that can be mitigated by hydration.[19] The uniqueness of the individual situation, the goals of care, the benefits and burdens of the proposed treatment, and the comfort of the patient must always be considered.[20]

Terminal Dehydration

Terminal dehydration refers to the process in which the dying patient's condition naturally results in a decrease in fluid intake. A gradual withdrawal from activities of daily living may occur as symptoms such as dysphagia, nausea, and fatigue become more obvious. Families commonly ask whether the patient will be thirsty as fluid intake decreases. Several studies have demonstrated that, although patients reported thirst, there was no correlation between thirst and hydration. Artificial hydration to relieve symptoms may be futile.[19] In addition, hydration has the potential to cause fluid accumulation, resulting in distressful symptoms associated with edema, ascites, nausea and vomiting, and pulmonary congestion. There is no evidence that rehydration prolongs life.[19] Nursing plays an important role in helping patients and family members to refocus on the natural course of the disease and that the patient's death will be caused by the disease, not by dehydration.

As the imminently dying person takes in less fluid, third-spaced fluids, clinically manifested as peripheral edema, ascites, or pleural effusions, may be reabsorbed. Breathing may become easier, and there may be less discomfort from tissue distention. In addition, as the person experiences dehydration, swelling is often reduced around tumor masses. Patients may experience transient improvements in comfort, including increased mental status and decreased pain. The family needs a careful and compassionate explanation regarding these temporary improvements and encouragement to make the most of this short but potentially meaningful time.

Dry Mouth

Dry mouth, a consistently reported distressing symptom of dehydration, can be relieved with sips of beverages, ice chips, or hard candies. Spraying normal saline into the mouth with a spray bottle or atomizer can also be helpful. (Normal saline is made by mixing one teaspoon of table salt in a quart of water.) Meticulous mouth care is essential and family members can be taught how to provide this care.

Medications

Medications unrelated to the terminal diagnosis are generally continued as long as their administration is not burdensome. When swallowing pills becomes too difficult, the medication may be offered in a liquid or other form if available. Continuing medications may be seen by some patients and families as a way of normalizing daily activities and therefore should be supported. Considerable tact, kindness, and knowledge of the patient and family are needed in assisting them to make decisions about discontinuing medications.

Medications that do not contribute to daily comfort should be evaluated on an individual basis for possible discontinuance. Medications such as antihypertensives, replacement hormones, vitamin supplements, iron preparations, hypoglycemics, long-term antibiotics, antiarrhythmics, and laxatives should be discontinued unless doing so would cause symptoms or discomfort. Special consideration should be given to the use of diuretics with patients with end-stage heart disease and corticosteroids in patients with neuropathic pain or for the treatment of increased intracranial pressure. The control or prevention of distressing symptoms is the guiding principle in the use of medications, especially in the final days of life. Resumption of the drug at any point is always an option if the need becomes apparent. Customarily, the only drugs necessary in the final days of life are analgesics, anticonvulsants, antiemetics, antipyretics, antisecretories, and sedatives.[21]

Implantable Cardioverter Defibrillator

Implantable cardioverter defibrillators (ICDs) are used to prevent cardiac arrest due to ventricular tachycardia or ventricular fibrillation. Patients with ICDs who are dying of another terminal condition or are withdrawn from antiarrhythmic medications may choose to have the defibrillator deactivated, or turned off, so that there will be no interference from the device at the time of death. If the patient has an ICD it is critical to confirm its deactivation if that is in keeping with the goals of care and the patient's religious beliefs. Routine screening for ICDs in out-of-institution care settings, like hospices, is suggested because of the high likelihood of preventable adverse events.[22,23] Deactivating the ICD is a simple, noninvasive procedure usually overseen by a cardiologist or an associated provider. The device is tested after it is turned off to ensure that it is no longer operational, and the test result is placed in the patient record. Patients and families often find this procedure important to provide assurance that death indeed will be quiet and easy when it does occur.

Renal Dialysis

Renal dialysis is a life-sustaining treatment, and as death approaches it is important to recognize and agree on its limitations.

Discontinuation of dialysis should be considered in the following cases:

- Patients with acute, concurrent illness, who, if they survive, will be faced with unwanted burden and disability as defined by the patient and family.
- Patients with progressive and untreatable disease or disability.
- Patients with severe dementia or severe neurological deficit.

Dialysis should not be used to prolong the dying process.[24] The time between discontinuing dialysis and death varies widely, from a matter of hours or days (for patients with acute illnesses) to days or a week or longer if some residual renal function remains.[24–25] Opening a discussion about the burden of treatment is a delicate task. There may be competing opinions among the patient, family, and staff about the tolerability or intolerability of continuing treatment. The nurse who sees the patient and family on a regular basis may be the best person to recognize the discrete changes in status. Validating these observations may open a much-needed discussion regarding the goals of care. The discussions and decisions surrounding discontinuation or modification of treatment are never easy. Phrases such as, "There is nothing more that can be done" or "We have tried everything" have no place in end-of-life discussions with patients and families. Always reassure the patient and family members—and be prepared to follow through—that you will stand by them and do all you can to provide help and comfort. This is essential to ensure that palliative care is not interpreted as abandonment.

Common Signs and Symptoms of Imminent Death and Their Management

The following signs and symptoms provide cues that death is only days away[1,9,26]:

- Profound weakness (patient is usually bedbound and requires assistance with all or most care).

- Gaunt and pale physical appearance (most common in persons with cancer if corticosteroids have not been used as part of treatment).

- Drowsiness and/or a reduction in awareness, insight, and perception (often with extended periods of drowsiness, extreme difficulty in concentrating, severely limited attention span, inability to cooperate with caregivers, disorientation to time and place, or semicomatose state).

- Increasing lack of interest in food and fluid with diminished intake (only able to take sips of fluids).

- Increasing difficulty in swallowing oral medications.

There are predictable sets of processes that occur during the final stages of a terminal illness associated with gradual hypoxia, respiratory acidosis, metabolic consequences of renal failure, and the signs and symptoms of hypoxic brain function.[1,9] These processes account for the signs and symptoms of imminent death and can assist the nurse in helping the family plan for the actual death.

During the final days, these signs and symptoms become more pronounced, and, as oxygen concentrations drop, new symptoms appear. Knowledge of the signs and symptoms associated with decreasing oxygen concentrations can assist the nurse in guiding the family as death nears.[26,27] As oxygen saturation drops below 80%, signs and symptoms related to hypoxia appear. Consideration of the individual perspective and associated relationships of the patient or family member, the underlying disease course trajectory, anticipated symptoms, and the setting of care is essential for optimal care at all stages of illness, but especially during the final days and hours.

Table 4.1 summarizes the physiological process of dying and suggests interventions for both patients and families. This list of symptoms and what to do about them may appear frightening, but knowing what to expect may reduce some of your anxiety about the approaching death. Each person approaches death in their own way, bringing to this last experience their own uniqueness. Our list of symptoms and suggested interventions is a map to the goal of a peaceful death. Like all maps, it shows many different routes to the same destination.

Table 4.2 describes the signs and symptoms of approaching death. You may see all of these symptoms or none. Death will come in its own time and its own way to each of us. It is important to remember that *dying is a natural process*.

Table 4.1 Symptoms in the Normal Progression of Dying and Suggested Interventions

Symptoms	Suggested Interventions
Early stage sensation/perception	• Interpret the signs and symptoms to the patient (when appropriate) and family as part of the normal dying process; for example, assure them the patient's "seeing" and even talking to persons who have died is normal and often expected.
• Impairment in the ability to grasp ideas and reason; periods of alertness along with periods of disorientation and restlessness are also noted.	
	• Urge family members to look for metaphors for death in speech and conversation (e.g., talk of a long journey, needing maps or tickets, or in preparing for a trip in other ways) and using these metaphors as a departure point for conversation with the patient.
	• Urge family to take advantage of the patient's periods of lucidity to talk with patient and ensure nothing is left unsaid.
	• Encourage family members to touch and speak slowly and gently to the patient without being patronizing.
	• Maximize safety; for example, use bedrails and schedule people to sit with the patient.
• Some loss of visual acuity.	• Keep sensory stimulation to a minimum, including light, sounds, and visual stimulation; reading to a patient who has enjoyed reading in the past may provide comfort.
• Increased sensitivity to bright lights while other senses, except hearing, are dulled.	• Urge the family to be mindful of what they say "over" the patient, because hearing remains present; also continue to urge family to say what they wish not to be left unsaid.
Cardiorespiratory	
• Increased pulse and respiratory rate.	• Normalize the observed changes by interpreting the signs and symptoms as part of the normal dying process and ensuring the patient's comfort.
• Agonal respirations or sounds of gasping for air without apparent discomfort.	
• Apnea, periodic, or Cheyne-Stokes respirations.	• Assess and treat respiratory distress as appropriate.

(continued)

Table 4.1 (Continued)

Symptoms	Suggested Interventions
• Inability to cough or clear secretions efficiently, resulting in gurgling or congested breathing (sometimes referred to as the "death rattle").	• Assess use and need for parenteral fluids, tube feedings, or hydration. (It is generally appropriate to either discontinue or greatly decrease these at this point in time.)
	• Reposition the patient in a side-lying position with the head of the bed elevated.
	• Suctioning is rarely needed, but when appropriate, suction should be gentle and only at the level of the mouth, throat, and nasal pharynx.
	• Administer anticholinergic drugs (transdermal scopolamine, hyoscyamine) as appropriate, recognizing and discussing with the family that they will not decrease already existing secretions.
Renal/Urinary	
• Decreasing urinary output, sometimes urinary incontinence or retention.	• Insert catheter and/or use absorbent padding.
	• Carefully assess for urinary retention, because restlessness can be a related symptom.
Musculoskeletal	
• Gradual loss of the ability to move, beginning with the legs, then progressing.	• Reposition every few hours as appropriate.
	• Anticipate needs such as sips of fluids, oral care, changing of bed pads and linens, and so on.
Late stage sensation/perception	
• Unconsciousness.	• Interpret the patient's unconsciousness to the family as part of the normal dying process.
• Eyes remain half open, blink reflex is absent; sense of hearing remains intact and may slowly decrease.	
	• Provide for total care, including incontinence of urine and stool.
	• Encourage family members to speak slowly and gently to the patient, with the assurance that hearing remains intact.
Cardiorespiratory	
• Heart rate may double, strength of contractions decrease; rhythm becomes irregular.	• Interpret these changes to family members as part of the normal dying process.
• Patient feels cool to the touch and becomes diaphoretic.	• Frequent linen changes and sponge baths may enhance comfort.

Table 4.1 (Continued)

Symptoms	Suggested Interventions
• Cyanosis is noted in the tip of the nose, nail beds, and knees; extremities may become mottled (progressive mottling indicates death within a few days); absence of a palpable radial pulse may indicate death within hours.	
Renal/Urinary	
• A precipitous drop in urinary output.	• Interpret to the family the drop in urinary output as a normal sign that death is near, usually between 24 and 72 hours away.
• Carefully assess for urinary retention; restlessness can be a related symptom.	

Care at the Time of Death, Death Rituals, and Facilitating Early Grieving

It is important to clarify specifically with family members what their desires and needs are at the time of death. Do they wish to be present? Do they know of others who wish to say a final goodbye? Have they said everything they wish to say to the person who is dying? Do they have any regrets? Are they concerned about anything? Do they wish something could be different? Every person in a family has different and unique needs that, unless explored, can go unmet. Family members recall the time before the death and immediately afterward with great acuity and detail. We only have the one chance to "get it right" and make the experience an individualized and memorable one.

Although an expected death can be anticipated with some degree of certainty, the exact time of death is often not predictable. Death may occur when no healthcare professionals are present. Dying people seem to determine the time of their own death—for example, waiting for someone to arrive, for a date or event to pass, or even for family members to leave—even if the leave-taking is brief. For this reason, it is crucial to ask family members who wish to be present at the time of death whether they have thought about the possibility they will not be there. This opens an essential discussion regarding the time of death and its unpredictability. Gently reminding family members of that possibility can assist them in preparing for any eventuality.

Family members' needs change around the time of death, just as the goals of care change. During this important time, plans are reviewed and perhaps refined. Special issues affecting the time of death, such as cultural influences, decisions regarding organ or body donation, and the need for autopsy, are also reviewed. Under US federal law, if death occurs in

Table 4.2 Signs and Symptoms of Approaching Death

1. *Withdrawal*—Physical and emotional, and increased sleep.	Natural process of withdrawing from everything outside of one's self, looking inward, reviewing one's self and one's life. Your loved one may turn inward, withdraw physically and emotionally. This occurs in an attempt to cope with the many changes that are occurring.
2. Reduced food and fluid intake.	Decreased *need* because body will naturally begin to conserve energy. Dehydration is a *natural comfort measure*, since the body systems cannot process fluids effectively. At no time should food/fluids be *forced*.
3. Confusion/Agitation can vary from mild to end-stage agitation, which may include trying to get out of bed, picking at covers, seeing things that are not apparent to us.	Talk calmly and assuredly. Keep lights on, use times when patient is alert for meaningful conversation. Music can be very calming. Medication often used to control this symptom.
4. Change in breathing patterns.	This is common. You may see irregular breathing: very rapid, very slow, and/or 10 to 30 seconds of no breathing at all (called apnea). These symptoms are very common and indicative of a decrease in circulation. It does not mean that your loved one is uncomfortable or struggling.
5. Oral secretions collect in back of throat causing noisy respiration.	Swallowing reflex may be absent. Patient may be breathing through the secretions.
	• This may be more uncomfortable for us as observers than for the patient experiencing it.
	• Elevate head of bed or turn patient on side.
6. Incontinence of urine and stool.	Reduced intake results in reduced output with darker color. Bedpads and diapers can be used to protect bed linens. Cleanse patient and change linens frequently to maintain comfort and protect skin.
7. Changes in skin temperature and color.	Decreased circulation can cause coolness and discoloration of skin. Use light covers, turn side to side frequently to maintain comfort and prevent skin breakdown (bedsores). Heating pads and electric blankets NOT recommended.

Hearing is the last sense to be lost, so the patient can hear all that is being said. This is a good time to say good-bye, reassure them that you will be all right even though you will miss them greatly. (You may tell them it's OK to "let go.") This permission is often helpful for a peaceful death.

How would you know death has occurred?

1. No breathing

2. No heartbeat or pulse

If you believe that death has occurred, call TRU Community Care 303-449-7740. Do not call 911 or the physician. We will come to your home to help you. (You may want to use the time until we arrive to say your last good-byes.)

Source: Courtesy of TRU Community Care, Colorado (formerly HospiceCare of Boulder and Broomfield Counties), Colorado, March, 2013.

a hospital setting, staff must approach the family decision-maker regarding the possibility of organ donation.[28] Although approaching family at this time may seem onerous, the opportunity to assist another is often comforting. Some hospital-based palliative care programs include information about organ donation in their admission or bereavement information. Importantly, the nurse can support the family's choice of death rituals, gently care for the body, assist in funeral planning, and facilitate the early process of grieving.

Determining That Death Has Occurred

Death often occurs when health professionals are not present at the bedside or in the home. Regardless of the site of death, a plan must be in place for who will be contacted, how the death pronouncement will be handled, and how the body will be removed. This is especially important for deaths that occur outside a healthcare institution. Death pronouncement procedures vary from state to state, and sometimes from county to county within a state. In some states, nurses can pronounce death; in others, they cannot. In inpatient settings, the organization's policy and procedures are followed. In hospice home care, generally the nurse makes a home visit, assesses the lack of vital signs, contacts the physician, who verbally agrees to sign the death certificate, and then contacts the funeral home or mortuary. Local customs, the ability of a healthcare agency to ensure the safety of a nurse during the home visit, and provision for "do-not-resuscitate" orders outside a hospital setting, among other factors, account for wide variability in the practices and procedures surrounding pronouncement of death in the home. Although practices vary widely, the police or coroner may need to be called if the circumstances of the death were unusual, were associated with trauma (regardless of the cause of the death), or occurred within 24 hours of a hospital admission.

The practice of actual death pronouncement varies widely. The customary procedure is to first identify the patient, then note the following:

- General appearance of the body.
- Lack of reaction to verbal or tactile stimuli.
- Lack of pupillary light reflex (pupils will be fixed and dilated).
- Absent breathing and lung sounds.
- Absent carotid and apical pulses (in some situations, listening for an apical pulse for a full minute is advisable).

Guidelines for documentation of death:

- Patient's name and time of call.
- Who was present at the time of death and at the time of the pronouncement.
- Detailed findings of the physical examination.
- Date and time of death pronouncement (either pronouncement by the nurse, or the time at which the physician either assessed the patient or was notified).

- Who else was notified and when—for example, additional family members, attending physician, or other staff members.
- Whether the coroner was notified, rationale, and outcome, if known.
- Special plans for disposition and outcome (e.g., organ or body donation, autopsy, special care related to cultural or religious traditions).

Care of the Body After Death

The care of the patient does not end with the death, but rather continues during the immediate postmortem period as the body is prepared for transport into the care of the funeral provider. Regardless of the site of death, care of the patient's body is an important nursing function. In gently caring for the body, the nurse can continue to communicate care and concern for the patient and family members and model behaviors that may be helpful as the family members continue their important grief work. Caring for the body after death also calls for an understanding of the physiological changes that occur. By understanding these changes, the nurse can interpret and dispel any myths and explain these changes to the family members. The scientific rationale for the postmortem procedure rests on the basis of the physiological changes that occur after death.[29] These changes occur at a regular rate depending on the temperature of the body at the time of death, the size of the body, the extent of infection (if any), and the temperature of the air. The three important physiological changes are rigor mortis, algor mortis, and postmortem decomposition.

Care of and respect for the body after death clearly communicate to the family that the person who died was indeed important and valued. Caring for the body after death can provide the needed link between family members and the reality of the death, recognizing that everyone present at the time of death and soon after will have a different experience and a different sense of loss. Many institutions no longer require nursing staff to care for patients after death or perform postmortem care. Further, there are few professional resources related to postmortem care and the most recent ones are not easily accessible.[30] Those available are largely found in the British nursing literature.[31–33] A recent analysis of postmortem policies in California hospitals found that the focus was primarily on legal procedures and the physical preparation of the body.[34] Postmortem care is clearly more than attention to the legal imperatives and physical care. A kind, gentle approach and meticulous attention to detail grounded in knowledge of the physiology of dying and death is imperative.

Rituals

Rituals that family members and others present find comforting should be encouraged. Rituals are practices within a social context that facilitate and provide ways to understand and cope with the contradictory and complex nature of human existence. They provide a means to express and contain strong emotions, ease feelings of anxiety and impotence, and provide structure in times of chaos and disorder. Rituals can take many forms—a brief service at the time of death, a special preparation of the body, as in the Orthodox Jewish tradition, or an Irish wake, where, after paying respect to the person who has died, family and friends gather to share stories, food, and drink. It is the family's needs and desires that direct this activity.

To facilitate the grieving process, it is often helpful to create a pleasant, peaceful, and comfortable environment for family members who wish to spend time with the body, according to their desires and cultural or religious traditions. Family members may engage in after-death care and ritual, for example, combing the hair or washing the person's hands and face. Parents can be encouraged to hold and cuddle their baby or child. Including siblings or other involved children in rituals, traditions, and other end-of-life care activities according to their developmental level is also important. During this time, family members are invited to talk about the family member who has died, and are encouraged to reminisce—valuable rituals that can help them begin to work through their grief. Parents may wish to clip and save a lock of hair as a keepsake. Babies may be wrapped snugly in a blanket. Many families choose to dress the body in a favorite article of clothing before removal by the funeral home. It should be noted that, at times, when a body is being turned, air escapes from the lungs, producing a "sighing" sound. Informing family members of this possibility is wise. If the eyes remain open they can often be closed by applying petroleum jelly to the eyelids.[35] Again, modeling gentle and careful handling of the body communicates care and concern on the part of the nurse and facilitates grieving and the creation of positive and long-lasting memories.

Postmortem care includes, unless an autopsy or the coroner is involved, removal of any tubes, drains, and other devices. In home care settings, these can be placed in a plastic bag and given to the funeral home for disposal as medical waste or simply double-bagged and placed in the family's regular trash. Placing a waterproof pad, diaper, or adult incontinence brief on the patient often prevents soiling and odor as the patient's body is moved and the rectal and urinary bladder sphincters relax. Occasionally families, especially in the home care setting, wish to keep the person's body at home, perhaps to wait for another family member to come from a distance and to ensure that everyone has adequate time with the deceased. If the family wishes the body to be embalmed, this is generally best done within 12 hours. If embalming is not desired, the body can, in most cases, remain in the home for approximately 24 hours before further decomposition and odor production occur. State laws vary on the amount of time a body can remain in the home and not be refrigerated. If the family wishes to have the body remain in the home, the nurse can suggest to the family that they adjust the temperature in the immediate area to a comfortable but cooler level and remove heavy blankets or coverings.[35] Be sure, however, to inform the funeral director that the family has chosen to keep the body at home a little longer. Finally, funeral directors are a reliable source of information regarding postdeath changes, local customs, and cultural issues. As the following case studies are reviewed, consider how the nurse interceded in a positive manner, mindful of the changing tempo of care and the changing patient and family needs, desires, and perspectives. Support of coworkers in providing after death care is important.[36]

Case Study: Tom, a 68-Year-Old Man With End-Stage Liver Disease

Tom, an unemployed veteran of the Vietnam War, had married twice in his life and divorced twice. Tom had two adult sons who live in nearby towns. He and his second wife were best of friends but "just could not live together." At the time of their divorce, he returned to his parents' home to live. Although that was initially disconcerting for his parents, he fulfilled an important role in helping them during the decline and death of his father. After the death of his father, his mother welcomed Tom's presence in the home even more. They were able to establish a respectful relationship that allowed each other to continue to function in their different communities of friends. Tom was a smoker and a former heavy drinker and, by all accounts, had a pretty unhealthy life. His mother and he were able to work out the details of their coexistence, basically tolerating each other's quirks. Tom's mother was grateful for some help around the house and yard, and Tom was grateful for a place to live.

Over time, Tom's mother noticed he was losing weight and had a slight yellowing of his skin. Tom would not answer when questioned about it, saying that he was fine. She persisted and urged him to go to a clinic and get it checked out. He resisted her "nagging," but promised he would see someone soon. He finally relented, made an appointment, and saw someone within a week. His provider told him she suspected cirrhosis and ordered more testing, including an abdominal ultrasound. Tom left the clinic without stopping at the lab or scheduling the ultrasound. He couldn't help thinking of a good friend who had died of liver disease a few years ago. He was frightened and didn't know where to turn.

Goals and Framework of Care

Upon Tom's return home from his first appointment, his mother asked, "so what is wrong and what is the plan?" Tom responded that he might follow up with a few tests, but wanted to wait and see. . . . His mother responded that she was really scared of what was going on, and hoped he would follow up as soon as possible. There was tension between the two, as both had different goals. The tension lasted for 2 weeks. Tom simply did not schedule appointments or plan to follow through. Then, one night, his mother found him collapsed on the bathroom floor. She called an ambulance, and he was admitted to the hospital, where he agreed to the previously ordered tests. He was diagnosed with end-stage cirrhosis.

After receiving the diagnosis, Tom refused consultation with a specialist. He just wanted to go home and get strong enough so he could hang out with his friends. He went home and was able to enjoy some time with his friends. After 2 weeks, he became confused and he collapsed again at home after vomiting frank blood. He was again admitted to the hospital, where esophageal varices were discovered; the bleeding stopped, and he received transfusions for his severe anemia.

Goals and Framework of Care

The shift in goals started at this time. Tom agreed to meet with a gastroenterologist, who evaluated the source of his bleeding and was able to ligate the source of the hemorrhage. Tom was also told he could lengthen his life by strictly adhering to the recommendations of diet and medications. Tom would not share his diagnosis with friends or his children. His mother decided she would. She told the staff simply, "I should tell them if he won't." Tom's former wife and children "stepped to the plate" quite well and talked to Tom openly about what they would like to do to help him and asked him to continue to dialogue with them.

Tom did experience a sense of control of his disease. Over the following 6 months, he was able to go hunting and fishing and help his mother with some of the projects that needed to be done on her house. At the end of 6 months, he again began to notice his stools were darker and again underwent ligation of his esophageal varices. He began exploring the chance of liver transplantation and, even though he was not considered an optimal candidate, met with the liver transplant center closest to home. He was hopeful this would work out—and started to work on stopping smoking. He was discouraged when he learned he was indeed not eligible for transplant but figured he would explore other options until he found a center that would be willing to put him on the transplant list.

Goals and Framework of Care

Suddenly there seemed to truly be a very large "elephant in the room." Death was the unspoken word. After a few days of this, his mother called his former wife and asked her if she would talk to Tom about his wishes. At her next visit, his former wife, Dixie, suggested that they speak with a lawyer, together. He agreed, and then next day, working together, Tom and Dixie "put his affairs in order." He also was able to talk with her about his preferences for care in the event (which to him seemed unlikely) he would not be able to make decisions for himself. He designated Dixie as the person he wanted to make decisions for him and completed the necessary documentation for the state they lived in.

Tom continued to contact transplant centers but became increasingly weak and fell several times while trying to get up out of his bed or chair. He also became delirious and began again to vomit frank blood. He returned to the hospital, where it was determined that he was in the end stages of liver failure and near death. Guided by his advance directive, the conversations he had with Dixie, and the prognostic estimation of the palliative care team, he was referred to a hospice program and transferred to an inpatient hospice facility. His delirium and pain were assessed and managed. Massive hemorrhage was anticipated and his mother and other visitors, including Dixie and his children, were prepared for the possibility. Additional medications were ordered and were readily accessible should hemorrhage occur. Five days later, he died quietly, about 10 minutes after his mother had left his bedside following an 8-hour vigil. Dixie later told his mother that dying alone was important to him.

His words, "I DID IT MY WAY." are on his gravestone, at his request.

4 Planning for the Actual Death

Critical Points

- Minimizing symptoms until they reach a critical point may be conscious decision of patients who have few remaining life goals.

- Open discussion of goals is controlled by the readiness of the patient.

- Recognizing the "moment" for the open discussion is critical. Encouraging family members to listen and "seize the moment" when it comes is an important family education point.

- Patients will do it their way. Helping them find their way is an important role of the nurse.

Case Study: Susan, a 30-Year-Old Woman With Breast Cancer

Susan was breastfeeding her first child, a son, 8 months old, when she noted a mass in her breast. She immediately saw her physician, who was not certain of the mass's relationship to lactation but ordered an ultrasound of the breast to be "on the safe side." The ultrasound was completed and was soon followed by a mammogram, biopsy, and diagnosis of Stage II breast cancer with one positive lymph node. Susan underwent a staging workup, surgery, and started chemotherapy within 3 weeks of noticing the breast lump. It was difficult for her to see past the positive lymph node; all discussions seemed to come back to the meaning of one positive node. Her anxiety was apparent during her interactions with care providers. Program staff worked to provide extra time and strong emotional support for her. Family and friends were present and expressed the desire to be ready to help at any time.

Goals and Framework of Care

Despite Susan's positive lymph node, the cancer was still considered "early" and very treatable. Susan successfully completed chemotherapy and radiation therapy and was set up for routine surveillance. She was encouraged to use the program's psychosocial resources to help her with any questions and particularly when her fears of recurrence and a dismal future seemed to immobilize her. Susan openly talked of what would happen if her cancer did reoccur. Who would assist her husband in raising her child? What would be important for her to leave her child? She was encouraged to think these things through, so she could have the appropriate discussions with her husband and then move forward as best she could. Slowly, she was able to do this. Susan focused on regaining her past lifestyle. She returned to community work on a part-time basis and often talked of the value of her work in helping others. She had a great sense of "giving back." Life seemed to settle for her, until one day when she called reporting a sudden onset of back pain. Bone scan and CT showed bone and early lung metastasis. Susan and her husband received imaging results together in the clinic and then opted to return the next day to speak with the medical oncologist.

Goals and Framework of Care

Together with her medical oncologist, Susan and her husband mapped out a plan for initial treatment. Although she was not eligible for clinical trials, she was interested in looking for any opportunity that would give her the best chance of quality time. She clearly stated her goal "to receive treatment that would buy as many days of 'quality time' that was available, defining quality time as being present, participating, and enjoying her son's daily life." Her goal had been well thought out. Susan started on chemotherapy. She responded well for 9 months, and had an "almost normal" life. When the second-line chemotherapy failed to control her disease, she agreed to the third-line chemotherapy. Although she tolerated the third line well, her disease progressed in spite of the treatment. Scans and lab work were not necessary to tell the staff that her liver function was rapidly declining. Ascites from her new liver metastasis complicated her comfort level and functional status. She agreed to hospitalization for symptomatic evaluation.

Goals and Framework of Care

During her admission to the hospital, Susan was offered a fourth-line chemotherapy regimen. After a quick discussion with her husband, she refused. She asked only that a plan for management of her discomfort be addressed, and that hospice be arranged for her. Susan said her good-byes to the staff. She was discharged with a home hospice program, stating she simply wanted to have the freedom to have her son with her to hug and cuddle without any restrictions or expectations. She died at home, surrounded by prepared, loving and caring family and friends, 48 hours later.

Critical Points

- Patients will often process their disease trajectory with minimal help other than the supportive, listening ears of their care providers.
- Patient fears are based in their reality, and we as care providers must not minimize or dismiss them.
- Patients who set clearly defined goals and are given the opportunity to share them with their care providers are generally observed to have a higher quality death experience for themselves, their family members, and the staff who care for them.

Summary

Caring for dying patients and their families is the essence of nursing care. It depends on the nurse having strong interpersonal skills and clinical knowledge—a combination of competence and compassion. By being present and using listening skills the nurse can provide the guidance to assure that the voice of the patient and family is heard through advance care planning, goals of care discussions, and the importance of cultural and religious practices as life draws to a close.

References

1. Twycross R, Lichter I. The terminal phase. In: Hanks G, Cherny NI, Christakis NA, Fallon M, Portenoy R, eds. Oxford Textbook of Palliative Medicine. 4th ed. Oxford: Oxford University Press; 2009:977–994.

2. Kehl KA, Kowalkowski JA. A systematic review of the prevalence of signs and symptoms of impending death and symptoms in the last 2 weeks of life. Am J Hosp Palliat Med. 2013;30(6):601–616.

3. Currow DC, Smith J, Davidson PM, Newton PJ, Agar MR, Abernathy AP. Do the trajectories of dyspnea differ in prevalence and intensity by diagnosis at end of life?: a consecutive cohort study. J Pain Symptom Manage. 2010;39:680–690.

4. Hendricks SA, Smakbrugge M, Hertogh CMPM, van der Steen JT. Dying with dementia: symptoms, treatment, and quality of life in the last week of life. J Pain Symptom Manage. 2013. Epub ahead of print. doi: 10.1016/j.jpainsymman.2013.05.015.

5. Moyer DD. Review article: terminal delirium in geriatric patients with cancer at end of life. Am J Hosp Palliat Care. 2011;28(1):44–51. doi: 10.1177/1049909110376755.

6. King S, Forbes K, Hanks GW, Ferro CJ, Chambers EJ. A systematic review of the use of opioid medication for those with moderate to severe cancer pain and renal impairment: a European Palliative Care Research Collaborative opioid guidelines project. Palliat Med. 2011;25(5):525–552.

7. Cambell ML, Yarandi HN. Death rattle is not associated with patient respiratory distress: is pharmacological treatment indicated? J Palliat Med. 2013;16(10):1255–1259. doi: 10.1089/jpm.2013.0122. Epub 2013 Sep 18.

8. Bailey FA, Williams BR, Goode PS, et al. Opioid pain medication orders and administration in the last days of life. J Pain Symptom Manage. 2012;44(5):681–691. doi: 10.1016/j.jpainsymman.2011.11.006. Epub 2012 July 4.

9. Ferris F. Last hours of living. Clin Ger Med. 2004;20:641–667.

10. Rogers C. On Becoming a Person: A Therapist's View of Psychology. Boston, MA: Houghton Mifflin; 1961.

11. National Consensus Project for Quality Palliative Care. Clinical Practice Guidelines for Quality Palliative Care. 3rd ed. Pittsburgh, PA: National Consensus Project for Quality Palliative Care; 2013. http://www.nationalconsensusproject.org. Accessed November 1, 2013.

12. Du Boulay S. Cicely Saunders: Founder of the Modern Hospice Movement. London, England: Hodder and Stoughton; 1984.

13. Ambuel B, Weissman D. Fast Fact and Concept #016: Conducting a Family Conference. 2nd ed. New York, NY: Center to Advance Palliative Care; 2009. https://www.capc.org/. Accessed July 18, 2015.

14. Osenga K, Cleary JF. Fever and sweats. In: Berger AM, Shuster JL, Von Roenn JH, eds. Principles and Practice of Palliative Care and Supportive Oncology. 3rd ed. New York, NY: Lippincott Williams & Wilkins; 2007:105–116.

15. Kazure HS, Roman SA, Sosa JA. Epidemiology and outcomes of in-hospital cardiopulmonary resuscitation in the United States, 2000–2009. Resuscitation. 2013;84(9):1255–1260. doi: 10.1016/j.resuscitation.2013.02.021. Epub March 5, 2013.

16. Kjorstad OJ, Haugen DF. Cardiopulmonary resuscitation in palliative care cancer patients. Tidsskr Nor Laegeforen. 2013;133(4):417–421. doi: 10.4045/tidsskr.12.0378.

17. Dunn H. Hard Choices for Loving People: CPR, Artificial Feeding, Comfort Care, and the Patient With a Life-Threatening Illness. 5th ed. Herndon, VA: A & A; 2009.

18. Zerwekh J. Do dying patients really need IV fluids? Am J Nurs. 1997;97:26–31.

19. Raijmakers NJH, van Zuylen L, Costantini M, et al. Artificial nutrition and hydration in the last week of life in cancer patients: a systematic literature review of practices and effects. Ann Oncol. 2011;22(7):1478–1486. doi: 10.1093/annonc/ mdq620.

20. Hospice and Palliative Nurses Association. HPNA Position Statement: Withholding and/or Withdrawing Life Sustaining Therapies. Pittsburgh, PA: Hospice and Palliative Nurses Association; 2011.

21. Working Party on Clinical Guidelines in Palliative Care. Changing Gear: Guidelines for Managing the Last Days of Life. London, England: National Council for Hospice and Specialist Palliative Care Services; 2010.

22. Fromme EK, Stewart TL, Jepperson M, Tolle SW. Adverse experiences with implantable defibrillators in Oregon hospices. Am J Hosp Palliat Care. 2011;28(5):304–309.

23. National Hospice and Palliative Care Organization. Position Statement on the Care of Hospice Patients with Automatic Implantable Cardioverter-Defibrillators. Arlington, VA: National Hospice and Palliative Care Organization; 2008.

24. Davison, SN, Rosielle DA. Fast Fact and Concept #207: Withdrawal of Dialysis: Decision-Making. New York, NY: Center to Advance Palliative Care; 2008. https://www.capc.org/. Accessed July 18, 2015.

25. Davison SN, Rosielle DA. Fast Facts and Concepts #208: Clinical Care Following Withdrawal of Dialysis. New York, NY: Center to Advance Palliative Care; 2008. https://www.capc.org/. Accessed July 18, 2015.

26. Hwang IC, Ahn HY, Park SM, Sim JY, Kim KK. Clinical changes in terminally ill cancer patients and death within 48 h: when should we refer patients to a separate room? Support Care Cancer. 2013;21:835–840. doi: 10.1007/s00520-012-1587-4.

27. Kehl KA, Kirchhoff KT, Finster MP, Cleary JF. Materials to prepare hospice families for dying in the home. J Palliat Med. 2008;11(7):969–972.

28. Department of Health and Human Services, Health Care Financing Administration. Medicare and Medicaid Programs; Hospital Conditions of Participation; Identification of Potential Organ, Tissue, and Eye Donors and Transplant Hospitals' Provision of Transplant-Related Data. Final rule. 63 Federal Register 119 (1998) (codified at 42 CFR §482.45).

29. Pennington EA. Postmortem care: more than ritual. Am J Nurs. 1978;75:846–847.

30. Caramanzana H, Wilches P. The final act of nursing care. J Contin Educ Nurs. 2012;43(7):295–296.

31. Beattie S. Hands-on-help: post-mortem care. RN. 2006;69(10): 24ac1–24ac4.

32. Higgins D. Clinical practical programs: carrying out last offices, Part 1—Preparing for the procedure. Nurs Times. 2008;104(37):20–21.

33. Higgins D. Clinical practical programs: carrying out last offices, Part 2—Preparation of the body. Nurs Times. 2008;104(38):24–25.

34. Smith-Stoner M, Hand MW. Expanding the concept of patient care: analysis of postmortem policies in California hospitals. Med Surg Nurs. 2012;21(6):360–366.

35. Tjaarda, Natasha, AAS, Licensed Funeral Director and Embalmer, Young's Funeral Home, Tigard, OR. Personal communication, June, 2013.

36. Olausson J, Ferrell BR. Care of the body after death: nurses' perspectives of the meaning of post-death patient care. Clin J Oncol Nurs. 2013;17(6):647–651.

Chapter 5

Cultural Considerations in Palliative Care

Polly Mazanec and Joan Panke

Key Points

- Culture consists of connections not separations.[1]
- Culture encompasses multiple components including race, ethnicity, gender, age, differing abilities, sexual orientation, religion, spirituality, and socioeconomic status.
- Quality palliative care requires attention to patient and family cultural values, practices, and beliefs.
- Palliative care staff need to cultivate cultural self-awareness and recognize how their own cultural values, beliefs, biases, and practices inform their perceptions of patients, families, and colleagues.

Culture consists of connections not separations.[1] It is a source of resilience for patients and families and plays an important role in the provision of palliative care.[2] The beliefs, norms, and practices of an individual's cultural heritage guide behavioral responses, decision-making, and actions.[3] Culture shapes how an individual makes meaning out of illness and death[3,4] This chapter defines culture and the complexity of its components as they relate to palliative care. It emphasizes the importance of recognizing not only how ones own values, practices, and beliefs may impact palliative care but also that patient and family values, beliefs, and practices should guide the plan of care.[5]

The National Consensus Project (NCP) Clinical Practice Guidelines for Quality Palliative Care[5] define the core concepts and structures for the delivery of quality palliative care. The guidelines comprise eight domains with corresponding criteria that reflect the depth and breadth of the specialty. Cultural aspects of care constitute one of the eight domains, emphasizing the central role that culture plays in providing strength and meaning for patients and families facing serious illness.[5] Within this domain, two overarching guidelines define culture and outline cultural competences for interdisciplinary team members (Box 5.1).

Box 5.1 Clinical Practice Guidelines for Quality Palliative Care—Cultural Aspects of Care

Guideline 6.1 The palliative care program serves each patient, family, and community in a culturally and linguistically appropriate manner.

Criteria:

- Definition of culture and cultural components
- Cultural identification of patient/family
- Assessment and documentation of cultural aspects of care
- The plan of care addresses the patient's and family's cultural concerns and needs.
- Respect for the patient's/family's cultural perceptions, preferences, and practices
- Palliative care program staff communicates in a language and manner that the patient and family understand and takes into account:
- Literacy
- Use of professional interpreter services and acceptable alternatives
- Written materials that facilitate patient/family understanding
- Respects and accommodates dietary and ritual practices of patients/families
- Palliative care staff members identify and refer patients/families to community resources as appropriate.

Guideline 6.2 The palliative care program strives to enhance its cultural and linguistic competence.

Criteria:

- Definition of cultural competence
- Valuing diversity in the work environment. Hiring practices of the palliative care program reflect the cultural and linguistic diversity of the community it serves.
- Palliative care staff cultivates cultural self-awareness and recognizes how their own cultural values, beliefs, biases, and practices inform their perceptions of patients, families, and colleagues.
- Provision of education to help staff members increase their cross-cultural knowledge and skills and reduce health disparities
- The palliative care program regularly evaluates and, if needed, modifies services, policies, and procedures to maximize its cultural and linguistic accessibility and responsiveness. Input from patients, families, and community stakeholders is integrated into this process.

Source: Adapted from National Consensus Project for Quality Palliative Care. Clinical Practice Guidelines for Quality Palliative Care 2013. www.nationalconsensusproject.org.

Case Study: Mrs. S, a 79-Year-Old Female With Congestive Heart Failure

Mrs. S is a 79-year-old female admitted to the hospital with decompensated congestive heart failure. She and her husband moved to the United States from China in the early 1970s and raised a daughter and son in the United States. Her 85-year-old husband is in good health. On morning rounds, the medical team spoke to the patient about her diagnosis, prognosis, likely disease course, and advance care planning concerns without any family present. The palliative care service was consulted in the afternoon to assist the primary team after the nurse found Mrs. S's husband helping her to dress and stating he was taking her to another hospital that would respect their ways.

Questions to Consider in This Case

1. What cultural issues are likely the basis for the conflict between the husband and medical team in this case?
2. What cultural, religious, and/or spiritual issues might impact decision-making?
3. Whom might the palliative team involve to assist in ascertaining religious or cultural aspects of care?
4. What are some techniques that the nurse and other health providers might use to both respect the patient's right to be involved in their care and ascertain what she wants to know and who makes decisions for this patient?

Increasing Diversity in the United States

As the United States becomes increasingly diverse, the range of treasured beliefs, shared teachings, norms, customs, and languages, challenges the nurse to both understand and respond to a wide variety of perspectives. The total US population in 2013 was estimated to be 317.3 million and was projected to cross the 400 billion mark by 2051.[6] (Population statistics from the US Census Bureau illustrate that cultural diversity is increasing among the five most common panethnic groups, which are federally defined as American Indian/Alaska Native, Asian/Pacific Islander, Black or African American, Hispanic, and White (Table 5.1).[7]

Asians and Hispanics are the nation's fastest-growing race or ethnic groups. Hispanics remain the second largest racial/ethnic group in the United States behind non-Hispanic Whites. Rates of growth in 2013 for other groups were as follows: Native Hawaiians and Other Pacific Islanders (climbing 2.3% to about 1.4 million), American Indians and Alaska Natives (rising 1.5% to a little over 6.4 million), and Blacks or African Americans (increasing 1.2% to 45 million) followed Asians and Hispanics in percentage growth rates.[8] Census projections suggest that by 2060 the combined minority groups, which currently make up 37% of the US population, will constitute the majority (57%).[7]

Table 5.1 Ethnic Groups, Census 2013	
White	197.8 million
Hispanic	54 million
Black or African American	45 million
Asian	19.4 million
American Indian/Alaskan Native	6.4 million
Hawaiian and Other Pacific Islanders	1.4 million
Source: https://www.census.gov/newsroom/releases/archives/population/cb14-118.html (assessed January 7, 2015)	

Diversity among age groups is also changing as the population ages. By 2060 the number of citizens aged 65 years and older will more than double and the number of the "oldest old," the 85-and-older age group, is expected to more than triple. It is likely that intergroup diversity will also increase, adding to the complexity of culturally competent care and the potential for cultural clashes. With the changes in cultural diversity in the US population come increasing diversity in the nursing workforce. Cultural beliefs and norms shape professional practice and may differ from the beliefs and norms of the patients and families for whom we care.

Culture Defined

Culture is the "learned, shared and transmitted values, beliefs, norms and life ways of a particular group that guide their thinking, decision, actions in patterned ways—a patterned behavioral response."[9]

Culture is shaped over time in a dynamic system in which the beliefs, values, and lifestyle patterns pass from one generation to another.[4] Culture is multidimensional, encompassing such components as gender, age, differing abilities, sexual orientation, religion, and socioeconomic factors (financial status, residency, employment, and educational level).[3] Each cultural component plays a role in shaping individual responses to life and in particular to serious illness and death.[3,4]

Components of Culture

A broad definition of culture recognizes the various subcultures within the dominant culture an individual may associate with that shape experiences and responses to any given situation. The nurse must be constantly aware that the culture of the healthcare system and the culture of the nursing profession, as well as personal beliefs, shape how he or she responds to interactions with patients, families, and colleagues.

Race

Race exists not as a natural category but as a social construct.[10] Any discussion of race must include the racism and disparities that have plagued society. Studies demonstrate the discrimination affecting persons of certain races regarding healthcare practices, treatment options, and hospice utilization.[11–14] Morbidity and mortality statistics point to serious gaps in access to quality care associated with racial disparities.[15] There is often distrust of the healthcare system. Memories of the Tuskegee syphilis study and segregated hospitals remain with older African Americans.[16] The combination of mistrust and numerous other variables influence medical decision-making and advance care planning and the perception of being discriminated against.[4,17–19] Evans and Ebere[13] recommend using a conceptual framework to explore causal mechanisms of disparities in care, including access to care, receipt of care, quality of care, barriers, usage, and costs of care, effectiveness, safety, timeliness, and patient centeredness.

Ethnicity

Ethnicity refers to "a group of people that share a common and distinctive racial, national, religious, linguistic, or cultural heritage."[19] The values, practices, and beliefs shared by members of the same ethnic group may influence behavior or response. Ethnicity has been identified as a significant predictor of end-of-life preferences and decision-making.[20] Currently, there are more than 100 ethnic groups and more than 500 American Indian Nations in the United States.[19] Ethnicity has been shown to influence use of hospice and palliative care service. Ethnic minority groups are less likely to use hospice services when compared with non-Hispanic Whites, and there has been little increase in hospice use among Black, Hispanic, or Asian populations in recent years.[17,21,22] In multigenerational families, some members may hold to traditional beliefs and practices of their ethnic community of origin. Other family members may have a bicultural orientation, moving between the family culture of origin to the host society, and others may have left their cultural roots and identify with the host society.[23,24] This can lead to cultural conflicts around certain palliative care concepts. However, many studies have demonstrated that regardless of race or ethnicity, all persons share common needs at the end of life: being comfortable, being cared for, sustaining or healing relationships, having hope, and honoring spiritual beliefs.[23–26]

Gender

Cultural norms dictate specific roles for men and women. The significance of gender is evident in areas such as decision-making, caregiving, and pain and symptom management. It is important to have an awareness of family dominance patterns and determine which family member or members hold that dominant role. In some families, decision-making may be the responsibility of the male head of the family or eldest son; in others, the eldest female may hold that responsibility. For example, those of Asian ethnicity who follow strict Confucian teaching believe that men have absolute authority and are responsible for family decision-making.[27] Discussing prognosis and treatment with a female family member is likely to increase family burden and distress and may result in significant clashes with the healthcare team.[3,23]

In addition to decision-making, cultural expectations exist regarding the responsibilities of caregiving. In many families, women have traditionally been expected to take on the role of caregiver when someone in the family is facing a serious illness. This responsibility, in addition to responsibilities at work and for children can be overwhelming for many, affecting their physical and emotional well-being. Research has demonstrated that female caregivers tend to experience greater caregiver burden, anxiety, and depression than male caregivers.[28,29] Support for family caregivers is an essential component of palliative care.

Age

Age has its own identity and culture.[3] Age cohorts are characterized by consumer behaviors, leisure activities, religious activities, education, and labor force participation.[24] The impact of a life-limiting illness on persons of differing age groups is often influenced by the loss of developmental tasks associated with that age group.[24,30] As the US population ages, the importance of addressing the unique needs of elders becomes more evident. Myths about the impact of age on pain management continue to exist, leading to unnecessary suffering.[26,31,32]

Differing Abilities

Individuals with physical disabilities or mental illness are at risk of receiving poor quality healthcare. Those with differing abilities constitute a cultural group in themselves and often feel stigmatized. This discrimination is evident in cultures where the healthy are more valued than the physically, emotionally, or intellectually challenged.[3] If patients are unable to communicate their needs, then pain and symptom management and end-of life wishes are not likely to be addressed. Additionally, this vulnerable population's losses may not be recognized or acknowledged, putting individuals at risk for complicated grief. Challenges to providing palliative care and hospice services to those with intellectual disabilities have been identified and include limited knowledge about palliative care among providers in residential facilities as well as a need for increasing the palliative care providers' knowledge about caring for patients with intellectual disabilities.[33]

Sexual Orientation

Sexual orientation may carry a stigma when the patient is gay, lesbian, or transgendered. In palliative care, these patients have unique needs because of the legal and ethical issues of domestic partnerships, multiple losses that may have been experienced as a result of one's sexual orientation, and unresolved family issues.

The US Supreme Court ruling in June 2015 legalizing same-sex marriage nationwide and according same-sex couples the same recognition as opposite-sex couples at the federal and state/territory level, should lessen some of the survivorship issues, financial concerns, and failure to acknowledge bereavement needs that have led to additional distress and complicated grief for the previously disenfranchised partner.[34,35] Unresolved family issues can make end-of-life complicated. Despite the new law, same-sex marriage remains controversial in some segments of society. The patient who is gay, lesbian, or transgendered may be estranged from his/her family of origin. Reconciliation with family, old friends, or children may be desired as the patient prepares for coming to the end of life, but may be challenging and distressing when family dynamics prohibit this opportunity for healing.[34]

Religion and Spirituality

Religion is the belief and practice of a faith tradition, a means of expressing spirituality. Spirituality, a much broader concept, is the life force that transcends our physical being and gives meaning and purpose.[30] Although religion and spirituality are complementary concepts, the terms are not interchangeable. An individual may be very spiritual but not practice a formal religion. In addition, those who identify themselves as belonging to a certain religion may not adhere to all the practices of that religion. As with ethnicity, it is important to determine how strongly the individual aligns with his or her identified faith and the significance of its practice rituals. Religious beliefs can significantly influence a person's decisions regarding treatment and care. These beliefs can be at the cornerstone for some people in decisions regarding continuation or discontinuation of life-prolonging treatments.[11,27] In addition, religious beliefs can strongly influence how patients and families understand illness and suffering.[4,11]

Chaplains or clergy from a patient's or family member's religious group are key members of the interdisciplinary palliative care team. Those who turn to their faith-based communities for support may find the emotional, spiritual, and other tangible support they need when dealing with a life-limiting illness.[13,25] Some community clergy are not trained in end-of-life care and may need assistance from the palliative care team in order to support the patient's spiritual journey. Spirituality is in the essence of every human being. It is what gives each person a sense of being, meaning, purpose, and direction.[36,37] It transcends the self to connect with others and with a higher power, independent of organized religion.[13,30,35] A sense of spirituality is often the force that helps transcend loss and suffering.[25,26,30] Spiritual distress can cause pain and suffering if not identified and addressed. Assessing spiritual well-being and attending to spiritual needs is essential to quality of life for patients and families confronting the end of life.

Socioeconomic Status

Socioeconomic status, place of residence, workplace, and level of education are important components of cultural identity and play a role in palliative care. Those who are socioeconomically disadvantaged face unique challenges when seeking healthcare. Financial costs, including pain medications, medical tests, treatments and drugs not covered by limited insurance plans, transportation, and childcare, add additional burden. Regardless of baseline financial status, however, an estimated 25% of families are financially devastated by a serious terminal illness.[3] Those who are educationally disadvantaged struggle to navigate the healthcare system and to find information and support. Access to services is challenging for some depending on their geographic location. For those living in rural areas, access to palliative care services is inadequate when compared with urban areas.[38] Only 57% of public hospitals, which serve those without healthcare insurance or those in rural areas, provide palliative care services.[39] Hospice services are also lacking, with 62%–92% of rural counties in selected states reporting no access to community-based hospice services.[40] A very vulnerable population with limited community resources is the undocumented immigrant. There are thought to be about 11.5 million undocumented immigrants in the United States (2012), most of whom are educationally and socioeconomically disadvantaged and living in the country with minimal access to healthcare.[41] Little is known about access to palliative care within this population.

Conducting a Cultural Assessment

There are many tools available to help with cultural assessment. These tools address the different components of culture. Doing a cultural assessment involves questions that necessitate the development of a trusting relationship. Using the skill of presence and active listening is more beneficial than using a standardized tool alone. Simple inquiries into patient and family practices and beliefs can assist the nurse in understanding needs and goals. Asking the patient and/or the family member to tell you about him/herself or the family and then listening to those narratives is powerful. The patient and family often give clues that trigger important questions to ask to clarify patient and family needs and goals (Box 5.2).

Selected Palliative Care Issues Influenced by Culture

Communication

Communication is the foundation for all encounters between clinicians, patients, and family members.[42] When the clinicians and the patient-family unit are from different ethnic or cultural backgrounds, relating news regarding serious illness or a poor prognosis can be challenging. Communication disparities may lead to poorer outcomes and reduced patient and family satisfaction.[4,43] Each individual brings his or her own cultural experiences and assumptions about the world, health, and illness to each new encounter. The establishment of a relationship with the clinician, where the clinician seeks to understand individual concerns of the patient and family provides a foundation for all future communication and decision-making.[23] Communication is an interactive, multidimensional process, often dictated by cultural norms, and provides the mechanism for human interaction and connection. Given the complexities of communicating diagnosis, prognosis, and progression of a life-limiting disease, there is no "one size fits all" approach.[44] Cultural assessments, including cultural norms related to communication, should occur early in the initial assessment, and findings should

Box 5.2 Key Cultural Assessment Questions

- Tell me a little bit about yourself (e.g., your family, your mother, father, siblings, etc.).

- Where were you born and raised? (If an immigrant, "How long have you lived in this country?")

- What language would you prefer to speak?

- Is it easier to write things down, or do you have difficulty with reading and writing?

- To whom do you go for support (family friends, community, or religious or community leaders)?

- Is there anyone we should contact to come to be with you?

- I want to be sure I'm giving you all the information you need. What do you want to know about your condition? To whom should I speak about your care?

- Whom do you want to know about your condition?

- How are decisions about healthcare made in your family? Should I speak directly with you, or is there someone else with whom I should be discussing decisions?

- (Address to patient or designated decision maker) Tell me about your understanding of what has been happening up to this point. What does the illness mean to you?

- We want to work with you to be sure you are getting the best care possible and that we are meeting all your needs. Is there anything we should know about any customs or practices that are important to include in your care?

- Many people have shared that it is very important to include spirituality or religion in their care. Is this something that is important for you? Our chaplain can help contact anyone that you would like to be involved with your care.

- We want to make sure we respect how you prefer to be addressed, including how we should act. Is there anything we should avoid? Is it appropriate for you to have male and female caregivers?

- Are there any foods you would like or that you should avoid?

- Do you have any concerns about how to pay for care, medications, or other services?

Death Rituals and Practices

- Is there anything we should know about care of the body, about rituals, practices, or ceremonies that should be performed?

- What is your belief about what happens after death?

- Is there a way for us to plan for anything you might need both at the time of death and afterward?

- Is there anything we should know about whether a man or a woman should be caring for the body after death?

- Should the family be involved in the care of the body?

be clearly documented and shared with all health providers involved in the care of the patient and family (Box 5.3).

One of the most important cultural communication assessments involves determining how information is shared within the family unit. Who is the decision maker, and with whom should information be shared? For example, relating a diagnosis or poor prognosis to the patient may go against some cultural norms. Listening to patient and family concerns, determining individual and group norms, and engaging in an ongoing dialogue about preferences will strengthen the relationship and show respect for the unique ways in which a family group functions.[45,46] If there is a language barrier, a professionally trained interpreter of the appropriate gender should be contacted. Family members should only act as interpreters in emergency situations.[3,5] When using an interpreter, all verbal communication should be directed to the patient/family rather than the interpreter. Ongoing clarification that information is understood is critical. Active listening is one of the most important communication techniques for the palliative care nurse to master. Nonverbal communication will give valuable information and insight into the emotional impact of what is being said.

Medical Decision-Making

Over the past 45 years in the United States, ethical and legal considerations of decision-making have focused on patient autonomy.[11,20] This focus replaced the more paternalistic approach, of decision-making as solely the physician's responsibility, with an approach that emphasizes a model of shared responsibility with the patient's active involvement.[17] The Patient Self-Determination Act of 1991 sought to further clarify and to protect an individual's healthcare preferences with advance directives.[47] The principle of respect for patient autonomy points to a patient's right to participate in decisions about the care he/she receives. Associated with this is the right to be informed of diagnosis, prognosis, and the risks and benefits of treatment to make informed decisions. Inherent in the movement for patient autonomy is the underlying assumption that all patients want control over their healthcare decisions. For some individuals, a rigid approach to patient autonomy may violate the very principles of dignity and integrity it proposes to uphold and may result in significant distress.[4,11]

This Western model of patient autonomy has its origin in the dominant culture, a predominantly white, middle-class perspective that does not consider the perspectives of diverse cultures.[4] In some cultures, patient autonomy may be viewed not as empowering but rather as isolating and burdensome for patients who are too sick to have to make difficult decisions.[4,11] Emphasis on autonomy as the guiding principle assumes that the individual, rather than the family or other social group, is the appropriate decision-maker.[4,17] However, in many non-European-American cultures, the concept of interdependence among family and community members is valued more than individual autonomy.[4,11,20] Cultures that practice family-centered decision-making, such as the Korean American and Mexican American cultures, may prefer that the family, or perhaps a particular family member rather than the patient, receive and process

Box 5.3 Culturally Competent Communication Skills and Best Practices for Palliative Care Clinicians

1. **Foster respect**. Baseline assessment and documentation should include primary language/dialect; determine need for professional interpreter services. Determine who is involved in giving/receiving information and decisions and how individuals prefer to be addressed.

2. **Perform person-centered interviews through active and reflective listening**. Hearing, understanding, retaining, analyzing, and evaluating information. Use information gleaned to guide future questions. Do not ask too many questions. Demonstrate active listening through an open body posture and eye contact (if culturally appropriate) and provide a private setting that is conducive to open communication. Reflect and restate essential content and determine other questions or concerns. Reaffirm intent to honor and respect individual/group decisions and plans.

3. **Provide presence**: Know your own beliefs and values and your level of comfort in engaging in conversations regarding illness and distress. Assist individuals to meet realistic goals when facing a serious illness, challenging situation, and/or uncertain future. Listen to the stories, life goals, and values. Pay attention to interpretation time, for example, how long it takes to make decisions, time needed to complete individual goals, imminence of death. Show empathy and compassion; be quiet/reflective during times of silence.

4. **Assess clinical knowledge of disease trajectories**. Assess and address distressing symptoms, side effects of treatment, and likely disease progression. Reaffirm goals of care and attempt the relief of symptoms and other concerns. Incorporate preferred healing practices and traditions. Discuss early access to hospice care to support goals as disease progresses.

5. **Determine learning styles and provide education to patient and family**. Determine any learning deficits. Provide educational materials in preferred language and/or arrange for professional interpreter when providing education. Do not overwhelm the patient and family with too much information at one time.

6. **Address nonverbal communication**. Nonverbal communication makes up the majority of communication between individuals. Assessing appropriate forms of nonverbal communication (for example eye contact) will assist in enhanced communication, demonstrate respect, and may avoid cultural conflict.

7. **Assess the individual's interpretation of what is important in life, what gives life meaning for them**. Understanding what is important to the individual and those closest to him/her will assist in individualizing the palliative care plan. Support patient's strengths and encourage the patient to maintain hope. Life review can help identify what gives life meaning.

(continued)

Box 5.3 (Continued)

8. **Assess and address religious and spiritual preferences and concerns**. It is important to understand the role a religious/faith community and spiritual beliefs and practice play in the patient's life. Consider including clergy and others that the individual/family identifies as key supports. Offer spiritual care (books, music, rituals, meditation, etc.) to enhance healing and peace.

9. **Demonstrate consideration of patient's privacy, decision-making strategies, and experience of loss and grief.** Early assessment of cultural issues related to beliefs about disclosure of diagnosis and decision-making preferences will ensure that care is given in ways that respect patient and family values. Observe for signs and symptoms of anticipatory or complicated grief and refer to appropriate interdisciplinary team members.

10. **Anticipate times when communication will be difficult**. Dealing with serious illness is often stressful. Be proactive by anticipating situations when communication may be difficult (i.e., breaking bad news, holding family meetings, and helping patients and family members communicate last wishes at the end of life). Utilize appropriate interdisciplinary team members to provide support to the patient and family during these difficult times.

Source: Adapted from C. Long. Ten best practices to enhance culturally competent communication in palliative care. Pediatr Hematol Oncol. 2011;33(suppl 2):S136–S139.

---

information.[11,13,48] For example, the traditional Chinese concept of "filial piety" requires that children are obligated to respect, care for, and protect their parents.[49] This obligation falls especially on the eldest son. Based on the values and beliefs of this culture, the son is obligated to protect the parent from the worry of a terminal prognosis. The principle of autonomy does allow for the patient to defer decision-making to others.

Although full disclosure may not be appropriate, it is never appropriate to lie to the patient. If the patient does not wish to receive information and/or telling the patient violates the patient's and family's cultural norms, the patient has the right not to receive the information. Some cultures believe that telling the patient he has a terminal illness strips away hope, causes needless suffering, and hastens death.[11,24] For example, imposing negative information, such as prognosis of a life-limiting illness, on the person who is ill is a dangerous violation of traditional Navajo values.[11] By asking how decisions are made and whether the patient wishes to be involved in both being told information or participating in the decision-making process, clinicians respect patient autonomy and honor individual beliefs and values.[46]

Discontinuation of Life-Prolonging Therapies

Attitudinal surveys evaluating initiating and terminating life-prolonging therapies have demonstrated differences among several ethnic groups. Research suggests that groups including African Americans, Chinese Americans,

Filipino Americans, Iranian Americans, Korean Americans, and Mexican Americans were more likely to start and to continue such therapies than were European Americans when such measures were felt by the healthcare team to be futile.[11,20,48,49] For families who believe that it is the duty of children to honor, respect, and care for their elders, allowing a parent to die may violate the principles of "filial piety" and bring shame and disgrace on the family.[49] Religious beliefs may also play a role in decisions about withholding or withdrawing medical interventions. For example, in the Christian Philippines, removing the ventilator is synonymous with euthanasia.[20] For those practicing Orthodox Judaism, the values that all life is precious and only God can decide our time to die are important, thus, agreeing to withdrawal of life-prolonging therapies may be in violation of their beliefs.[50] In both examples, involving a priest or rabbi may help the families and the healthcare team integrate religious tenets into the culturally appropriate plan of care. Because many ethical conflicts arise from differences in patients', families', and providers' values, beliefs, and practices, it is critical that individual members of the healthcare team be aware of their own cultural beliefs, understand their own reactions to the issue, and be knowledgeable about the patients' and families' beliefs in order to address the conflict.[3,46]

Meaning of Food and Nutrition

Across cultures, there is agreement that food is essential for life to maintain body function and to produce energy.[27] Food serves another purpose in the building and maintaining of human relationships. It is used in rituals, celebrations, and rites of passage to establish and maintain social and cultural relationships with families, friends, and others. Culturally appropriate foods may be used to improve health by groups who have strong beliefs about particular foods and their relationship to health.[27] Because of food's importance for life and life events, a loss of desire for food, and subsequent weight loss and wasting, can cause suffering for both the patient and family. Families often struggle when the patient is no longer taking in any nourishment or fluids, fearing that the patient will "starve to death" or suffer from dehydration. It is imperative that the healthcare team understand the meaning attached to food and nutrition when discussions regarding the benefit and burden ratio of providing artificial nutrition and hydration for an imminently dying patient take place. Exploring alternative ways in which the family can care for the patient in ways that are meaningful to them and reflect individual beliefs, values, and preferences is important. The Hospice and Palliative Nurses Association Position Statement on Artificial Nutrition and Hydration in Advanced Illness can assist the nurse in understanding the benefits and burdens associated with this medical intervention.[51]

Pain and Symptom Management

Pain is a highly personal and subjective experience. Culture plays a role in the experience of pain, the meaning of pain, and the response to pain. The meaning of pain varies among cultural groups. For some, pain is a positive response that demonstrates the body's ability to fight against disease or the dying process. For others, pain signifies punishment and its value lies in the patient's ability to withstand the suffering and work toward resolution and peace.[18,52] Strong beliefs about expressing pain and expected pain behaviors exist in every culture.[52] Pain assessment should be culturally appropriate, using terms that describe pain intensity across most cultural groups. "Pain," "hurt," and "ache" are words commonly used across cultures. Pain-rating scales have been translated into numerous languages.[53] A consistent approach to assessing pain and pain relief in a particular patient should be used by all those caring for the patient and documented in that manner. Racial, ethnic, age, and gender biases in pain management have been identified and documented.[31,52] Studies of gender variations in pain response have identified differences in sensitivity and tolerance to pain as well as willingness to report pain.[52] Compared with men, women are more likely to report pain and have a lower pain threshold and tolerance in experimental settings.[52] Underidentification and undertreatment of pain is a well-recognized phenomenon in elder care.[54] Studies show that Hispanics, African Americans, and females are less likely to be prescribed opioids for pain or may be unable to fill opioid prescriptions depending on community access to pharmacies.[18]

Like pain, symptoms described by patients receiving palliative care may have meanings associated with them that reflect cultural values, beliefs, and practices. Assessment and management of symptoms such as fatigue, dyspnea, depression, nausea and vomiting, and anorexia/cachexia should be addressed within a cultural framework. For example, some cultural groups may be hesitant to disclose depression because it is considered a sign of weakness; instead it may be referred to as a "tired state."

Incorporating culturally appropriate nondrug therapies may improve the ability to alleviate pain and symptoms. Herbal remedies, acupuncture, and folk medicines should be incorporated into the plan of care if desired, keeping in mind that certain nondrug approaches, such as hypnosis and massage, may be inappropriate in some cultures.[46]

Death Rituals and Mourning Practices

The loss of a loved one brings sadness and upheaval in the family structure across all cultures. Each culture responds to these losses through specific rituals that assist the dying and the bereaved through the final transition from life.[30,46] Rituals may begin before death and may last for months or even years after death. Respecting these rituals and customs will impact on the healing process for family members following the death and leave a positive lasting memory of the loved one's end-of-life experience. For example, dying at home is especially important for Hmong American elders who follow traditional beliefs.[55] The family may consult a shaman to perform a ceremony to negotiate with the "God of the sky" to extend life. Additional ceremonies follow. Request for an autopsy or organ donation at the time of death is inappropriate because of the belief that altering the body will delay reincarnation. After the death, there is often much wailing and caressing of the body. The family prepares for an elaborate funeral with rituals to ensure that the loved one will "cross over" and continues with ceremonies for days following the funeral to make sure the soul joins its ancestors.[55]

The tasks of grieving are universal: to accept the reality of the loss, to experience pain of grief, to begin the adjustment to new social and family roles, and to withdraw emotional energy from the dead individual and turn it over to those who are alive.[56] The expressions of grief, however, may vary significantly among cultures. Recognizing normal grief behavior (vs. complicated grief) within a cultural context demands knowledge about culturally acceptable expressions of grief.[3,56]

Case Study: Mr. M, a 62-Year-Old Male With Stage IV Non-Small-Cell Lung Cancer

Mr. M. is a 62-year-old Vietnam War Veteran who came to the Veteran's Affairs Medical Center for an evaluation of a cough, fatigue, weight loss, and pain in his right hip. He had not sought medical care for these symptoms, which had been going on for over 3 months. The outpatient oncology team was consulted for a new diagnosis of Stage IV non-small-cell lung cancer at the same time the palliative care service was called to assist with his care. Despite increasing pain in his hip and later in his chest wall, he refused any pain medication other than ibuprofen. He repeatedly stated, "I am a tough Marine, I can take it, this is nothing compared to what some of my buddies went through in Nam." He confided in the chaplain that, "I deserve this, after all the people I hurt and killed in the war-this is payback." His anxiety and depressive symptoms worsened as the disease progressed. His wife and adult daughters were extremely distressed witnessing his suffering.

Questions to Consider in This Case

1. What cultural issues may be contributing to the challenges of pain and symptom management for Mr. M.?[57,58]
2. What spiritual issues need to be addressed for a peaceful death?
3. What are some techniques that the nurse and other healthcare providers might use to help the family as well as the staff with moral distress surrounding poor pain control?

Cultural Competence

Cultural competence refers to a dynamic, fluid, continuous process of awareness, knowledge, skill, interaction, and sensitivity.[59,60] The term is controversial.[3] Some social scientists suggest that the term "cultural humility" is more acceptable than cultural sensitivity or cultural competence when trying to provide culturally appropriate care.[60] Cultural competence is an ongoing process, not an endpoint or something to be mastered.[23] It is more comprehensive than cultural sensitivity, implying not only the ability to recognize and respect cultural differences but also to intervene appropriately and effectively. Integrating cultural considerations into palliative care requires awareness of how one's own values, practices, and

Box 5.4 Web Resources for Acquiring Knowledge About Cultural Issues Affecting Healthcare

Cross Cultural Health Care Program (CCHCP): www.xcul.ture.org

CCHCP addresses broad cultural issues that impact the health of individuals and families in ethnic minority communities. Its mission is to serve as a bridge between communities and healthcare institutions.

Diversity Rx: http://www.diversityrx.org

This is a great networking website that models and practices policy, legal issues, and links to other resources.

EthnoMed: http://ethnomed.org/

The EthnoMed site contains information about cultural beliefs, medical issues, and other related issues pertinent to the healthcare of recent immigrants to the United States.

Fast Fact & Concept #78; Cultural Aspects of Pain Management: https://www.capc.org. This website contains many "fast facts" regarding palliative care. Number 78 addresses important cultural considerations and provides assessment questions when working with patients in pain.

Fast Fact & Concept # 216: Asking About Cultural Beliefs in Palliative Care: https://www.capc.org. This resource offers a framework for assessing patient and family cultural needs by taking a "cultural history."

Office of Minority Health: https://minorityhealth.hhs.gov

This website has training tools for developing cultural competency.

Transcultural Nursing Society: http://www.tcns.org

The society (founded in 1974) serves as a forum to promote, advance, and disseminate transcultural nursing knowledge worldwide.

beliefs influence care.[57] Exploring one's own beliefs will raise an awareness of differences that have the potential to foster prejudice and discrimination and limit the effectiveness of care.[3,46] Exploring answers to the same cultural assessment questions used for patients and families increases self-awareness (Box 5.2).

Cultural guides, literature, and web-based resources are available to assist the nurse in acquiring knowledge about specific groups.[27] Box 5.4 lists several useful web-based resources and serves as a starting point for gaining more information.

Summary

Culture fundamentally shapes how an individual makes meaning out of illness, suffering, and death. It also influences how a person interacts with the healthcare system. Different cultures embrace different values and ideas about healthcare, how decisions are made, and the dying process. Nursing attributes that are essential to culturally sensitive care include flexibility, empathy, a nonjudgmental approach, language facility, and competence in approaches to sharing information about decision-making. Cultural practices become increasingly important at end of life.

References

1. Fuentes C. Myself With Others: Selected Essays. London, England: Deutsch; 1988.

2. Coyle N. Introduction to palliative nursing care. In Ferrell BR, Coyle N, Paice, J. eds. Textbook of Palliative Nursing. 4th ed. New York, NY: Oxford University Press; 2015:3–10.

3. End-of-Life Nursing Education Consortium (ELNEC). http://www.aacn.nche.edu/elnec/. Accessed February 23, 2015.

4. Kagawa-Singer M. Impact of culture on health outcomes. Pediat Hematol Oncol. 2011;33(suppl 2):S90–S95.

5. National Consensus Project for Quality Palliative Care. Clinical Practice Guidelines for Quality Palliative Care. 3rd ed. Pittsburgh, PA: National Consensus Project for Quality Palliative Care; 2013.

6. US Census Bureau. Census Bureau Projects US Population of 317.3 Million on New Years Day 2014. Washington, DC: US Census Bureau; 2013. http://www.commerce.gov/blog/2013/12/30/census-bureau-projects-us-population-3173-million-new-year%E2%80%99s-day. Accessed February 24, 2015.

7. US Census Bureau. US Census Bureau Projections Show a Slower Growing, Older, More Diverse Nation a Half Century From Now. Washington, DC: US Census Bureau; 2012. https://www.census.gov/newsroom/releases/archives/population/cb12-243.html. Accessed February 27, 2015.

8. US Census Bureau. Census Bureau Reports June 26, 2014. Washington, DC: US Census Bureau; 2014. http://www.census.gov/newsroom/releases/archives/population/cb14-118.html. Accessed February 6, 2015.

9. Leininger M. Quality of life from a transcultural nursing perspective. Nurs Sci Quart. 1994;7:22–28.

10. Koffman J, Crawley L. Ethnic and cultural aspects of palliative care. In: Hanks G, Cherney NI, Christakis NA, Fallon M, Kaasa S, Portenoy RK, eds. Oxford Textbook of Palliative Medicine. 4th ed. New York, NY: Oxford University Press; 2011:141–150.

11. Johnstone MJ, Kanitsaki O. Ethics and advance care planning in a culturally diverse society. J Transcult Nurs. 2009;20:405–416.

12. Cohen LL. Racial/ethnic disparities in hospice care: a systematic review. J Palliat Med. 2008;5:763–767.

13. Evans BC, Ebere U. Psychosocial, cultural, and spiritual health disparities in end-of-life and palliative care: where we are and where we need to go. Nurs Outlook. 2012;60:370–375.

14. Hulme, PA. Cultural considerations in evidence-based practice. J Transcult Nurs. 2010;21:271–280.

15. Smedley B, Stith A, Nelson A. Unequal treatment: confronting racial and ethnic disparities in health care (Report of the Institute of Medicine). Washington, DC: National Academy Press; 2003.

16. Brandon DT, Isaac LA, LaVeist TA. The legacy of Tuskegee and trust in medical care: is Tuskegee responsible for race differences in mistrust of medical care? J Natl Med Assoc. 2005;97:951–956.

17. Bullock K. The influence of culture on end-of-life decision making. J Soc Work End Life Palliat Care. 2011;7:83–98.

18. Anderson KC, Green CR, Payne R. Racial and ethnic disparities in pain: causes and consequences of unequal care. J Pain. 2009;10:1187–1204.

19. Office of Minority Health: National Center on Minority Health and Health Disparities. http://www.ncmhd.nih.gov. Accessed June 29, 2013.

20. Manalo, MF. End-of Life decisions about withholding or withdrawing therapy: medical, ethical, and religio-cultural considerations. Palliat Care: Res Treat. 2013;7:1–5.

21. Mazanec PM, Daly BJ, Townsend A. Hospice utilization and end-of-life decision making of African Americans. Amer J Hosp Palliat Med. 2010;27:560–566.

22. The Science of Compassion: Future Directions in EOL and Palliative Care; Executive Summary. Bethesda, MD: National Institute of Nursing Research (NINR); 2011:1–18.

23. Wittenberg-Lyles E, Goldsmith J, Ferrell BR, Ragan SL. Communication in Palliative Nursing. New York, NY: Oxford University Press; 2012:59–92.

24. Long CO. Ten best practices to enhance culturally competent communication in palliative care. Pediatr Hematol Oncol. 2011;33(suppl 2):S136–S139.

25. Prince-Paul MJ. Relationships among communicative acts, social well-being, and spiritual well-being on the quality of life at the end of life in patients with cancer enrolled in hospice. J Palliat Med. 2008;11:20–25.

26. Ferrell B, Coyle N. The Nature of Suffering and the Goals of Nursing. New York, NY: Oxford University Press; 2008.

27. Spector R. Cultural Care: Guides to Heritage Assessment and Health Traditions. 7th ed. Upper Saddle River, NJ: Pearson Education; 2009.

28. Northouse L, Williams A, Given B, McCorkle R. Psychosocial care for the caregivers of patients with cancer. J Clin Oncol. 2012;30(11):1227–1234.

29. Otis-Green S, Juarez G. Enhancing the social well-being of family caregivers. Semin Oncol Nurs. 2012;28(4):246–255.

30. Sherman D. Culture and spirituality as domains of quality palliative care. In: Matzo M, Sherman D, eds. Palliative Care Nursing: Quality Care to the End of Life. 4th ed. New York, NY: Springer; 2015:92–127.

31. Krok JL, Baker TA, McMillan SC. Age differences in the presence of pain and psychological distress in younger and older cancer patients. J Hosp Palliat Nurs. 2013;15:107–113.

32. Soltow D, Given BA, Given CW. Relationship between age and symptoms of pain and fatigue in adults undergoing treatment for cancer. Cancer Nurs. 2010;33(4):296–303.

33. Stein, GL. Providing palliative care to people with intellectual disabilities: services, staff knowledge, and challenges. J Palliat Med. 2008;11:1241–1249.

34. Rawlings D. End-of-life care considerations for gay, lesbian, bisexual, and transgender individuals. Int J Palliat Nurs. 2012;18:29–34.

35. Higgins A, Glacken M. Sculpting the distress: easing or exacerbating the grief experience of same-sex couples. Int J Palliat Nurs. 2009;15(4):170–176.

36. Puchalski CM, Ferrell BR, Virani R, et al. Improving the quality of spiritual care as a dimension of palliative care: the report of the consensus conference. J Palliat Med. 2009;12(10):885–904.

37. Puchalski CM, Ferrell BR. Making Health Care Whole: Integrating Spirituality Into Patient Care. West Conshohocken, PA: Templeton; 2010.

38. Lynch S. Hospice and palliative care access issues in rural areas. Amer J Hosp Palliat Med. 2012;30:172–177.

39. Morrison RA, Meier DE. Report Card: America's Care of Serious Illness: A State by State Report Card on Access to Palliative Care in Our Nation's Hospitals. New York, NY: New York Center to Advance Palliative Care; National Palliative Care Research Center; 2011.

40. Madigan EA, Wiencek CA, Vander Schrier AL. Patterns of community-based end-of-life care in rural areas of the United States. Policy Polit Nurs Pract. 2009;10(1):71–81.

41. Heflt PR. To keep them from injustice: reflections on the care of unauthorized immigrants with cancer. J Oncol Pract. 2012;8(4):212–214.

42. Dahlin CM. Wittenberg E. Communication in palliative care: an essential competency for nurses. In: Ferrell BR, Coyle N, Paice J, eds. Oxford Textbook of Palliative Nursing. 4th ed. New York, NY: Oxford University Press; 2015:81–109.

43. Butow P, Bella M, Goldstein D, et al. Grappling with cultural differences: communication between oncologists and immigrant cancer patients with and without interpreters. Patient Educ Couns. 2011;84:398–405.

44. Williams SW, Hanson LC, Boyd C, et al. Communication, decision making, and cancer: what African Americans want physicians to know. J Palliat Med. 2008;11:1221–1226.

45. Barclay JS, Blackhall LJ, Tulsky JA. Communication strategies and cultural issues in the delivery of bad news. J Palliat Med. 2007;10:958–977.

46. Foley H, Mazanec P. Culture and considerations in palliative care. In Panke JT, Coyne P, eds. Conversations in Palliative Care. 3rd ed. Pittsburg PA: Hospice and Palliative Nurses Association; 2011:157–163.

47. Federal Patient Self-Determination Act 1990, 42 U.S.C. 1395 cc(a).

48. Hsiung YY, Ferrans CE. Recognizing Chinese Americans' cultural needs in making end-of-life treatment decisions. J Hosp Palliat Nurs. 2007;9:132–140.

49. Taxis JC. Mexican Americans and hospice care: culture, control, and communication. J Hosp Palliat Nurs. 2008;10:133–161.

50. Schultz M, Bar-Sela G. Initiating palliative care conversations: lessons from Jewish bioethics. J Supp Onc. 2013;11(1):1–7. http://dx.doi.org/10.1016j.suponc.2012.07.003. Accessed June 20, 2013.

51. HPNA Position Statement on Artificial Nutrition and Hydration in End-of-Life Care. http://www.hpna.org/pdf/Artifical_Nutrition_and_Hydration_PDF.pdfHPNA. Accessed June 24, 2014.

52. Wadner LD, Scipio CD, Hirsch AT, Torres CA, Robinson ME. The perception of pain in others: how gender, race, and age influence pain expectations. J Pain. 2012;13:220–227.

53. McCaffery M, Pasero C. Pain: Clinical Manual. 2nd ed. St. Louis, MO: Mosby; 1999.

54. Reynolds KS, Hanson LC, Henderson M, Steinhauser KE. End-of-life care in nursing home settings: do race or age matter? Palliat Support Care. 2008;6:21–27.

55. Gerdner LA, Yang D, Tripp-Reimer T. The circle of life: end-of-life care and death rituals for Hmong-American elders. J Gerontol Nurs. 2007;33:20–29.

56. O'Mallon MO. Vulnerable populations: exploring a family perspective of grief. J Hosp Palliat Nurs. 2009;11:91–98.

57. Hallarman L, Kearns C. The military history as a vehicle for exploring end-of-life care with veterans. J Palliat Med. 2008;11:104–105.

58. Bixby KA, Bateman J. Caring for veterans. In Panke JT, Coyne P, eds. Conversations in Palliative Care. 3rd ed. Pittsburg PA: Hospice and Palliative Nurses Association; 2011:283–294.

59. Campinha-Bacote J. A model and instrument for addressing cultural competence in health care. J Nurs Educ. 1999;38:203–207.

60. Nyatanga B. Cultural competence: a noble idea in a changing world. Intern J Palliat Nurs. 2008;14:315.

Appendix

Self-Assessment Test Questions

Nessa Coyle

Questions

1. A 51-year-old home care patient has end-stage alcoholic cirrhosis. He has a history of physical and emotional abuse of his wife and daughters. He is receiving 360 mg of sustained-release morphine every 12 hours with 100 mg of immediate-release morphine every 1 hour prn. He consistently rates his pain at 8 on a scale of 0 to 10. After adjusting the pain medications, which of the following would be the MOST appropriate action?

    A. Obtain an order for an antianxiety medication.
    B. Discuss placement in a long-term care facility.
    C. Consider a plan to address unresolved relationship issues.
    D. Arrange for a volunteer to provide respite care for the wife.

2. In the home of a prospective patient, the hospice nurse has just explained that hospice serves those who have a limited life expectancy. The spouse then becomes extremely angry, stating that their physician has not told them that the patient is dying. At this point, the nurse's BEST response is to

    A. inquire what the physician has told the spouse.
    B. counsel the spouse to call the physician.
    C. assess the patient's physical and functional status.
    D. explain the patient's disease process.

3. A 45-year-old woman is widowed, has breast cancer with brain metastases, and lives with her five young children and her sister. She has been optimistic about her prognosis, but now has intermittent confusion. In an attempt to protect her children, she has not shared information about her condition. All of the following are appropriate for the plan of care EXCEPT

    A. Assessing the children's understanding of the condition.
    B. Encouraging the patient to set up guardianship for her children.
    C. Assessing her sister's understanding of the situation.
    D. Focusing care on the patient and letting her handle her family issues.

4. A nurse is making an initial home visit with a patient and the family. The family recently moved to the United States from Asia. Which of the following MOST likely characterizes the use of social touch in the care of this patient and family?

    A. Social touch by staff members may be viewed as inappropriate.

    B. Treatment will not be valued unless social touch is also involved.

    C. Social touch with the patient is acceptable, but not with the family.

    D. Social touch is only acceptable between patients and staff of the same gender.

5. A 39-year-old father is dying, and his wife is caring for him. His two young children are not allowed to be in his room. How should the interdisciplinary team proceed INITIALLY?

    A. Discuss reasons for the children's exclusion with the parents.

    B. Respect the parents' wishes and refer the children to a grief group.

    C. Arrange for spiritual and social work counseling for the family.

    D. Have a volunteer stay with the children for a few hours every day.

6. A child whose mother has just died asks if her mommy will be back in time for her birthday. The hospice nurse should explore the child's understanding of death related to

    A. causality.

    B. universality.

    C. irreversibility.

    D. nonfunctionality.

7. A woman's husband died 9 months ago after a painful illness. The woman's daughter notifies the bereavement coordinator that her mother is still suffering. Which of the following statements would indicate that she is experiencing an abnormal grieving process?

    A. "I visit his grave site every Sunday."

    B. "I'm just no good to anyone any more."

    C. "It's hard to cook for just one person."

    D. "Sometimes I feel so angry at my husband."

8. Six weeks after admission to hospice, an elderly wife is no longer able to care for her husband. They have no relatives. Neighbors are helpful, but also elderly. The couple wants to remain at home. Which of the following should the nurse recommend?

    A. social work referral

    B. nursing home placement

    C. daily home health aide visits

    D. volunteer visits 3 times a day

9. The nurse arrives to admit a patient to home hospice. She discovers that the caregiver has not given any medications, although written

discharge instructions and the medications were in the home. The nurse should FIRST

A. prepare a written medication schedule.
B. evaluate the caregiver's cognitive ability.
C. reeducate the caregiver about the medication regimen.
D. set up the medications in a daily pill organizer.

10. Which of the following is the MOST appropriate action if a nurse observes a patient verbally abusing his wife?

A. Alert the social worker.
B. Involve a volunteer for respite.
C. Notify adult protective services
D. Counsel the patient on self-control.

Answers

1. C
2. A
3. D
4. A
5. A
6. C
7. B
8. A
9. B
10. A

Index

Page numbers followed by f, t, or b indicate figures, tables, or boxes, respectively.

123